Karen Stolman, M.D., a U.S. board-certified dermatologist, is an assistant professor of dermatology at the University of Utah School of Medicine. She has been practicing dermatology for over twenty years. She is also the author of two skincare websites. Dr. Stolman lives in Utah with her husband and two sons.

This book is dedicated to the dermatologist who mentored me first—my father, Lewis Stolman, M.D.

To my beautiful mother, Cynthia Stolman, Ph.D., who taught me at a young age to achieve and to never listen to those who doubted me.

To my patients, who cheered me on and inspired me to write and teach.

And to my always supportive family: Eric, Caden, and Grant.

Karen Stolman, M.D.

30 – DAY SKIN FIX

Rapid Ways to Better Skin

AUSTIN MACAULEY PUBLISHERS™

LONDON • CAMBRIDGE • NEW YORK • SHARJAH

Ordering Information:
Quantity sales: special discounts are available on quantity purchases by corporations, associations, and others. For details, contact the publisher at the address below.

Publisher's Cataloging-in-Publication data
Stolman M.D., Karen
30-Day Skin Fix

ISBN 9781645361848 (Paperback)
ISBN 9781645361855 (Hardback)
ISBN 9781645366065 (ePub e-book)

Library of Congress Control Number: 2020901871

www.austinmacauley.com/us

First Published (2020)
Austin Macauley Publishers LLC
40 Wall Street, 28th Floor
New York, NY 10005
USA

mail-usa@austinmacauley.com
+1 (646) 5125767

I would like to express my deepest gratitude to my co-workers and staff at the University of Utah for all their support and belief in me. I also wish to thank my sister, Lara Stolman Watzky J.D., for always being there and lending me her wisdom.

Introduction
Read Me First!

Have you been freaking out because your skin is looking terrible and you have just a month or less until you need to look your best? Maybe it's your graduation, prom, or wedding? A reunion, birthday, or holiday? Maybe you have more than thirty days, maybe you don't? Then this book is for you.

Your skin doesn't hide unless you hide. There are simple and scientifically proven things that you can do that will improve most skin problems quickly, whether it is acne, eczema, rosacea, or other bad skin problems. I am a board-certified Dermatologist, practicing for over twenty years, and have helped thousands of people clear up their skin quickly. At your typical dermatology clinic visit, there is not enough time to go into all the tricks we know to improve your skin. In this book, I will present to you these tricks as very easy steps to quickly fix your bad skin. I will address common skin problems like rashes, eczema, acne, rosacea, and skin wounds and how to heal them faster than you ever imagined.

There is no guarantee that your skin will improve in thirty days if you follow these steps and you should not follow a step that contains anything to which you think you are allergic. A little secret among dermatologists: most of our treatments will take effect within thirty days, and can rescue your skin quickly. Many of them can be done at home without a prescription, but I will occasionally name options that are from the doctor's office or prescription pad that can be done as well. This book is intentionally short, and is not a text book. I do not want you to get frustrated or bored trying to fix your skin. I do get into details about some skin problems where I know it will clear up a common question or confusion. My hope is that you pick up some valuable knowledge so you can take better command of your skin, and feel less like you are at the mercy of your skin. You do not need to have a skin problem right now to benefit from reading this book. There are plenty of everyday tips to help you maintain beautiful, healthy skin all your life.

Do not wait any longer. It is time to read how to fix your skin in thirty days or less!

Chapter 1

You Must Cleanse

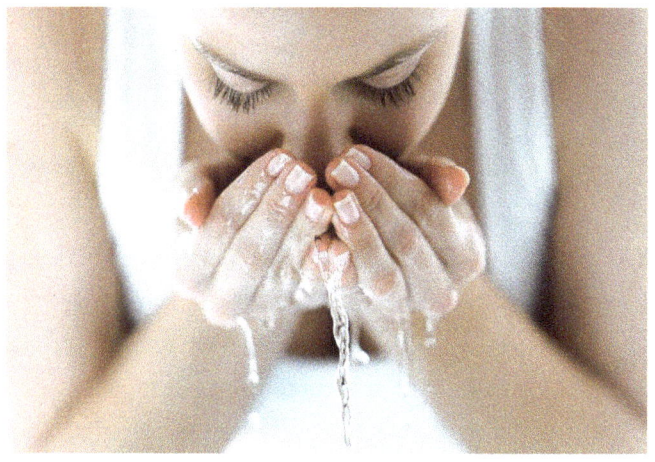

I know that your mother already told you to wash your face every day. She probably even said that not washing your face enough is why you have acne or bad skin. That is not entirely true, as acne is more complicated than just bad hygiene and involves skin cell turnover, sebaceous gland activity, hormones, heredity, diet, and more. Nevertheless, gentle cleansing of the skin is crucial to having healthy, good skin, whether acne or not. Dermatologists figured out in the last couple decades how best to wash your face, how many times a day, and with what. Keep reading and you will find out.

It is scientifically proven that in order to have healthy skin washing the face should be done gently with mild cleansers twice a day with fingertips or hands, not harsh soaps or detergents.

When we do not cleanse in this way oil, grime, residue, and dead skin cells may accumulate on our skin causing dermatitis and/or acne. People with bad cleansing habits or poor hygiene tend to have more acne, dermatitis, and skin infections. People who over-cleanse their skin also may suffer from more dermatitis and skin infections. This is because harsh cleansing can inflame the skin. It can make it more vulnerable to infection and even, clog pores.

The skin rash I see the most in clinic is triggered or worsened from under-cleansing your face. This common rash is dandruff of the face (seborrheic dermatitis). Second, after dandruff, would be yeast acne. These are both oily skin problems that can be better controlled with regular cleansing. A rash that I see from over-cleansing the face is eczema or worsened acne. Gently cleansing twice a day with a mild cleanser as I described above is the safest way to accomplish proper face cleansing.

You do not need microdermabrasion, spinning brushes, or other fancy cleansing systems, which may even cause inflammation and more skin problems in some people. Gritty sandy cleansers are also not necessary. One of the reasons I am not a fan of home microdermabrasion is that I have seen people spread infections on their skin and worsen rather than improve. Some cleansers contain exfoliants and mild acids like: salicylic, alpha-hydroxy, and glycolic.

These exfoliating cleansers are helpful for certain types of skin problems such as acne and oily skin. I prefer these exfoliating cleansers or even home chemical peels to home microdermabrasion because they will give similar results but without the risk of spreading infection. Just keep in mind, anything that exfoliates the skin will make you more susceptible to sun damage and sunburn.

Retinoids: Why You Cannot Live Without Them

If you are determined to exfoliate to clear pores, then a retinoid cream or gel can do that just as well as home microdermabrasion or exfoliating cleansers. Besides exfoliating, retinoids control sebaceous oil to improve acne, fade brown discolorations, and thicken collagen and elastin in the skin. We can help improve wrinkles and thin scars or stretch marks with this last property of retinoids. Retinoids are now available over-the-counter without a prescription or can be prescribed by your dermatologist in stronger strengths. Retinoids are so important and helpful to maintaining healthy skin that I have heard my dermatologist colleagues' joke: "Everyone and their mother should be on a retinoid." Beware, a retinoid may take at least thirty days to kick in fully and see improvement in the skin. Sometimes when we wait for the retinoid to kick in, we feel like we look worse. I like to describe this side effect of retinoid use as a 'purge.' You may see a temporary increase in whiteheads or surface pimples, even if you don't normally have those, as the retinoid does its work in clearing out your skin. If you need to do something faster and cannot wait 4

– 6 weeks for the retinoid 'purge' to clear, then don't start a retinoid. In order to clear out pores or comedones rapidly, you can see your doctor for comedone extraction and a gentle chemical peel up to at least two weeks before your event.

To Tone or Not to Tone

Growing up reading Seventeen magazine, I thought 'Sea Breeze' and 'Ten O Six' were going to clear my skin and cure my acne. They smelled like they would. The truth is, traditional astringents, like alcohol, or oil-control toners are best for very oily skin and may be too drying for normal or dry skin. Instead, modern toners we now see in the market are meant for balancing pH of our skin so we are less likely to get infections, rashes, and breakouts. Stress, hormone changes, and some diet choices may change the pH of our skin, which in turn can result in irritated, inflamed, or broken-out skin. Look for gentle toners that restore normal pH for these benefits and apply daily up to twice a day after cleansing. Dermatologists now believe that unhealthy skin pH may be an important cause or trigger of acne and skin rashes. Not only do toners help correct skin pH, but gentle cleansers and moisturizers may fix your skin pH as well. You can see Chapter 5 for more information about pH and the skin.

Chapter 2

Calm and Stop the Inflammation

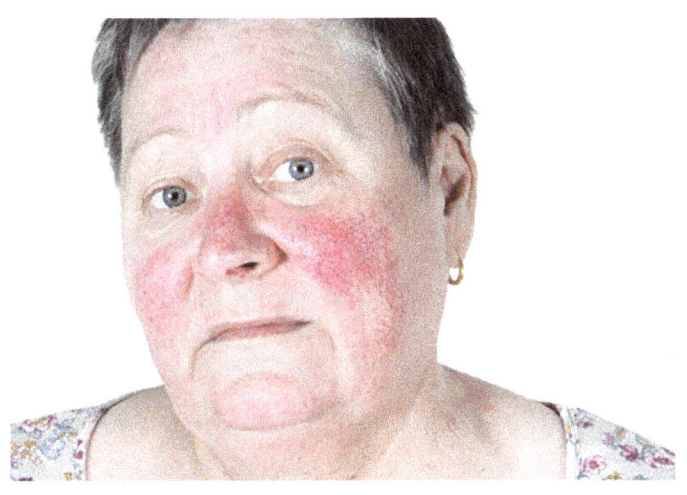

What Is Inflammation?

When your skin looks bad and angry, there usually is inflammation. Inflammation underlies the most common skin diseases, like eczema, acne, rosacea, and even some less common skin disorders like psoriasis. The woman in the picture above with very rosy cheeks has rosacea, which is marked by a tendency to flush easily. While we do not yet know all the causes of rosacea, we can see evidence of inflammation and vasospasm or blood vessel spasm. There are also theories about the increased presence of mites on the skin in rosacea.

What is inflammation in the skin and what does it look like? Inflammation of the skin usually looks and feels like redness, swelling, itching, and sometimes pain. When inflammation occurs in the skin, it may be because there was either inflammation inside the body elsewhere or there was a direct attack on the skin to trigger the inflammation.

More Common Diseases That May Cause Inflamed Skin

Dermatologists will use the term dermatitis to refer to inflamed skin. In inflamed skin with psoriasis, there can be inflammation in other places in the body like the joints and heart and blood vessels, and not just the skin. Here I will give you an overview of some more common dermatitis rashes, some of which you may have or know about, and others you may not have and not care about. I will do a quick overview and try not to bore you, but just enough information so you understand what it means to have inflamed skin and how we can manage it at home.

Some people get rashes from their perfume or jewelry. This is a type of contact dermatitis. Sometimes, it is an actual allergy to nickel and we call it an allergic contact dermatitis. Other times it is just irritation and not an actual allergy causing the dermatitis and we call this an irritant contact dermatitis. For example if you are wetting and washing your hands a lot or over-washing, then you may get an irritant dermatitis. It could be worse right under where your ring or watch sits. Inflammation in the skin can also be caused by bad habits like picking or scratching. Some people with nickel allergy will also react to nickel in food. If you suspect you have nickel allergy, I recommend you avoid nickel-rich foods. You can find a list of foods to avoid, go to the ContactDerm.Org[1] website's link given in the footnote.

People with eczema have inflamed skin frequently, and tend to be allergy-prone and their skin may be more reactive. Asthma, allergies, and hay fever are associated with eczema. Food allergies are found more often in people with more severe eczema but do not explain all the flare-ups. When you have eczema, your skin pH tends to be too alkaline, so measures I discussed earlier on how to fix pH with toners, cleansers, and moisturizers tend to be helpful. As to why the skin is inflamed in eczema, it will be discussed in more detail in Chapter 4.

Rosacea is a common cause of pink/red inflamed cheeks, nose, and chin. You can tell if you have rosacea if the redness is made up of visible small veins and you tend to flush or blush easily. All skin types, fair and dark, may get rosacea, but it does seem to be more common in fair skin types. Many people with rosacea get pimples and confuse their skin bumps with acne. A key difference between a rosacea pimple and an acne pimple is that the acne pimple always starts as a 'comedone' or blackhead or whitehead, whereas the rosacea pimple just pops out pink or red or pus-filled.

---

[1]https://www.contactderm.org/files/public/Patient%20Handouts/ZZ%20NICKEL.pdf

The most important triggers of redness and rosacea to avoid are sun, alcohol, and heat, but many people will flare-up with certain foods. Spicy foods, alcoholic drinks, or foods, temperature-hot foods, and the following foods could trigger rosacea as per rosacea.org:

Liver
Yogurt
Sour cream
Cheese (except cottage cheese)
Chocolate
Vanilla
Soy sauce
Yeast extract (bread is OK)
Vinegar
Eggplant
Avocados
Spinach
Broad-leaf beans and pods,
Including lima, navy, or pea
Citrus fruits, tomatoes, bananas,
red plums, raisins, or figs
Foods high in histamine

To battle the redness at home, you must avoid irritants or exfoliators on your skin like home microdermabrasion devices or rotating brushes or abrasive cleansers. In general, with rosacea, your skin is more sensitive and you should avoid heavily medicated cleansers meant for acne. You should also avoid chemical peels. Choose gentle, hypoallergenic skin cleansers and moisturizers.

It is important that everyone know about a super common condition called seborrheic dermatitis, which is also known as dandruff. It may occur on and around the face, ears, or scalp. Just about everyone gets this. No one is spared from dandruff. It is worse in children and the elderly. While most of us know when we have dandruff in the scalp, many of us confuse dandruff of the face with other things like eczema or acne. That's because dandruff on the face can look like small pimples or red rashes with flaking or peeling. The trick that most dermatologists know to tell dandruff on the face from other rashes is that dandruff will almost only occur where there are lots of active sebaceous glands. This is on the T-zone. In addition, dandruff is believed to be triggered by yeast, and this pityrosporum type of yeast can often be seen with a black light or Wood's lamp. If you have a black light at home, you may be able to see the dandruff-causing yeast as coral pink glitter. I will delve a little deeper into discussing dandruff in Chapter 4.

Another common cause of inflammation of the skin is infection. My dermatology colleagues and I have been seeing a lot more of staph and strep infections of the skin in my office ever since the internet and, now, TV trend to watch people popping their zits. Most people think they can do it at home but fail and make matters worse by spreading the infection. The mistakes they usually make is over squeezing and failing to properly incise the top of the abscess, which is best done surgically by a doctor, anyway. There are controlled ways of draining a swollen pimple or cyst and this is best done with sterile instruments with the experience and skill of the dermatologist. If you follow the tips I give in this book for daily care of your skin, you will be less likely to get problems like this.

Burns from Sun, Chemicals, or Heat

Burns inflame the skin, so to halt the pain and damage from the burn and prevent discoloration or scarring, it is important to stop the inflammation. Immediately after sustaining a burn, begin with application of cool water or cool compresses. Apply natural herbal anti-inflammatories like pure aloe vera or calendula, then apply a bland, fragrance-free, hypoallergenic moisturizer. When choosing aloe vera or calendula, avoid manufactured brands that contain perfumes and dyes. Other anti-inflammatories found in some lotions that you can apply to a burn are niacinamide and licorice root extract. You may also apply a hydrocortisone cream to help calm the inflammation. Hydrocortisone should not be used beyond a week on the face to avoid side effects like acne. All these anti-inflammatory ingredients can be applied together for more results. In the first few days following a burn, it is also helpful to take an oral anti-inflammatory like aspirin or ibuprofen. It should be taken twice to three times a day for a few days until the pain, redness, and swelling subside.

Starting in the second to third week or when peeling, blister, pain, swelling, and redness in the burn have subsided, it is best to treat the wound with antioxidants. Burns oxidize the cells in our skin, which may cause pre-cancerous changes. Oxidation is at the root of aging and cancer formation. With all the many choices of antioxidants, topical and oral, there are plenty of options to reverse the damaging oxidation of burns. I recommend taking an oral multivitamin and applying a topical antioxidant, serum, or lotion. There are numerous skin care brands that offer these antioxidants but verify that the product has been proven clinically with scientific studies. It is also best to choose an antioxidant topical product that has multiple antioxidants mixed in one. Use the antioxidants to your wound for at least a month for best results.

Shaving Bumps and Consequences

Shaving can be a risky endeavor. The most common problems from shaving are: irritation, cuts, wounds, acne, and folliculitis. Folliculitis is redness and swelling, which is centered on the hair follicle and can be just inflammation or infected. It is seen on beards, necks, armpits, groins, buttocks, legs, and arms. There are some steps that can be taken to avoid problems with shaving.

If shaving the face, using a higher quality electric shaver is less likely to give bumps. When shaving the body anywhere below the neck, using razors with extra moisturizing strips are safest. Always shave with warm water. Shaving the body in a warm shower with a gentle soap is safest. Avoid shaving creams as they tend to have too many irritating additives. If you have done all these things and are still struggling with shaving bumps, then it may be time to see the dermatologist and make sure you do not have an infection or other dermatitis. Infections tend to spread beyond where the razor travelled, whereas direct irritation from the razor is usually limited to the path of the razor.

If you are needing a hair removal solution and you are fed up with shaving and its hazards, then consider laser hair removal. Laser hair removal is best done on darker hair with lighter skin. The lasers have trouble seeing lighter colored hair or hair that does not contrast well with the background skin. Darker skin types can also be treated with certain types of hair removal lasers. Usually YAG lasers are used for hair removal in darker skin. For permanent thinning with laser hair removal, treatments are repeated six to seven times six weeks apart. Yes, permanent thinning, not permanent removal, as with today's technology we do not see 100% permanent removal of all the hairs with lasers.

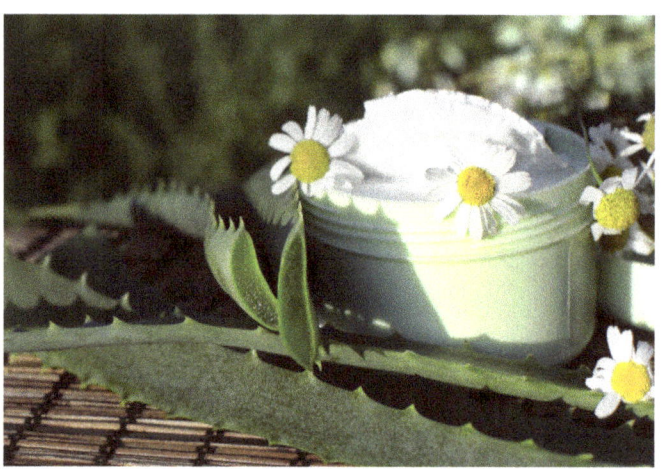

Home Topical Remedies for Inflamed Skin

Mostly every skin disease is treated by the dermatologist with control of unwanted inflammation in mind. Even some very inflamed skin diseases will improve with anti-inflammatory remedies that can be purchased or found easily without a prescription. Topical steroid creams are the first-line remedy for inflamed skin that is not caused by infection. In general, they are safe to use up to a few days on the face and up to a few weeks on the rest of the skin for inflammation or rashes. The main side effects and concerns with overuse are acne and thinning of the skin with stretchmark formation. The following are natural topical ingredients to help calm inflamed skin: aloe vera, calendula, niacinamide, rose water, licorice root extract, green tea, feverfew, colloidal oatmeal, allantoin, gingko biloba, and chamomile. It is helpful to have these ingredients at hand, as I explained earlier. The topical steroid creams cannot be safely used for prolonged periods of time. In addition, thermal spring water and pH-balancing gels, serums, or sprays can also be done at home to calm the inflamed skin. Beware of the new prescription anti-redness gels (brimonidine and others), as they can produce rebound redness and side effects like irritation of the skin, and even drowsiness and low blood pressure. There are stories of people over-applying this medicine and ending up in the ER with dizziness.

Home Oral Remedies for Inflamed Skin

Now let's discuss some oral options to do at home without a prescription. If you think you have an allergy rash, then taking an antihistamine like Benadryl, Claritin, Zyrtec, or Allegra or similar may be helpful to calm your rash and your itch. If you have an acne or rosacea flare-up, sometimes, just taking an ibuprofen or aspirin can help calm the inflammation but not everyone tolerates these due to stomach upset or its blood-thinning effects. Oral supplements that contain ginger, turmeric, zinc, white willow bark, and omega 3and 6 oils may also help calm your inflamed skin.

Home LED

Another exciting home treatment option for inflammation in the skin are LED light devices. LED lights have been shown to calm inflammation in the skin. If inflamed skin is a regular event for you, you may want to consider investing in one of these home devices. They do need repeating and regular use but are pain-free, sometimes relaxing, and convenient.

Time to Go to the Doctor

If you are not improving with these measures at home, then you may benefit from a proper diagnosis with the dermatologist and a prescription which may include topical or oral steroids or oral antibiotics. There are some gentle lasers and light treatments that can be done in the doctor's office as well, which may heal certain inflammatory skin problems faster.

Chapter 3

Fade the Brown Spots

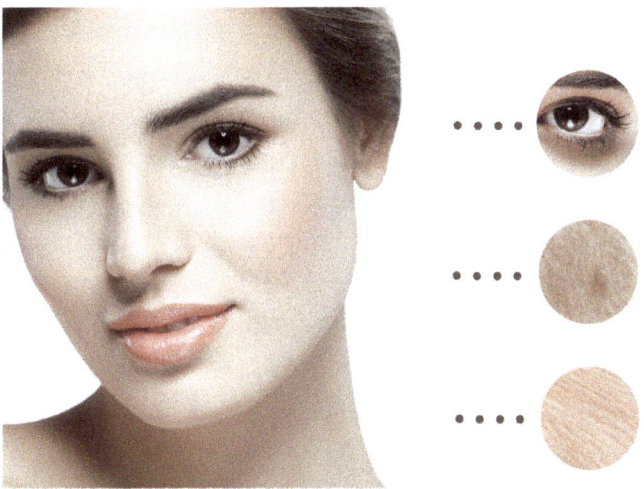

Now that you have calmed the inflammation after getting through Chapter 2, you may still be panicking about brown discoloration, marks, or scars.

Browns spots, marks, and scars are more challenging to fade when we just have thirty days or less but it is possible to improve them very quickly. The first rule is no picking. When you pick or squeeze things on the skin, you are bringing more problem inflammation to the skin and this delays healing and worsens marks and scars. If you already picked before reading this book, then, hopefully, you have improved since reading Chapter 2, or go back and read it. If your skin has healed to the point where it is no longer raw, then you may try a brown spot or scar treatment.

Home Topical Remedies

A little secret...cortisone creams can fade color, so could be tried, but should not be continuously applied to the face for more than one week or to the body for more than three weeks. Dermatologists like to mix cortisone with tretinoin (retinoids) and with hydroquinone (bleaching agent) as a more powerful topical mixture to fade brown spots. This combination can be powerful and simulated at home with store-bought versions of these ingredients. Usually, there is some improvement with twice-daily use of this combination cream just one month, though best results may take three to four months. Other home brown spot fading ingredients that can be found without a prescription include: kojic acid, tranexamic acid, retinol, licorice root extract, and niacinamide. Retinol and 'growth factor or peptide' creams can be very helpful for thinned scars or stretch marks. I recommend you note these ingredients and look for them online or bring a list to the pharmacy store as a reference. All of these home remedies will be helpful at thirty days but for the most benefit can be used for four to six months. After that, you may plateau in your degree of improvement.

Doing It at Home with a Topical Prescription

Your dermatologist may prescribe a topical retinoid or hydroquinone cream to fade brown. The retinoid can also be used to improve texture in thinned scars or stretch marks. These prescriptions are helpful but not necessarily superior to the other at-home treatments I discussed above. Retinoids are now more available over-the-counter without a prescription. Differin 0.1% gel was the first prescription retinoid to transition to over-the-counter in recent years. Retinols can be purchased without a prescription and are often similar in strength to the lowest prescription strength of a retinoid. Whether it is prescription ingredients or over-the-counter to be consistent and to be persistent is the key to success.

Oral Remedies

Polypodium leucotomos

Oral supplements containing Polypodium leucotomos extract, such as 'Heliocare' have been clinically proven to improve the blotchy brown skin of melasma. In addition, this herbal extract has been shown to help prevent skin damage from ultraviolet light exposure.

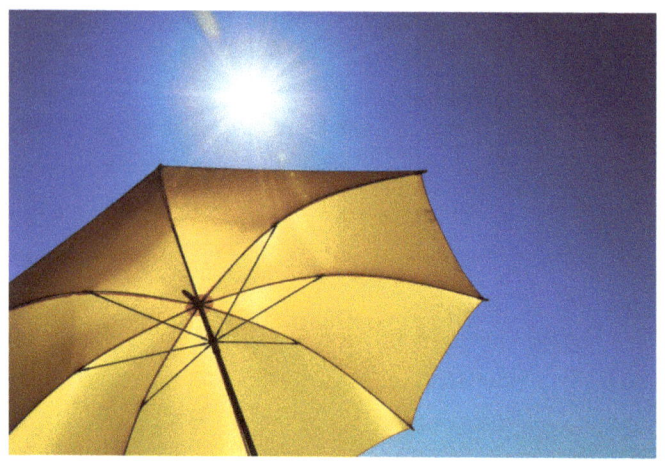

People who have frequent outdoor jobs or activities and are concerned about their excessive sun exposure may benefit from taking such a supplement.

Tranexamic Acid

Your dermatologist can prescribe an oral medication called tranexamic acid to improve your melasma. This medication has been shown to be helpful for improving even deep or dermal melasma but it is unclear how long lasting that benefit will be. In addition, some people may not be good candidates for this medication. If you have a history of an abnormal blood clot or clotting disorder or take any other medications that increase clotting risk, you may not be a candidate to take tranexamic acid orally. You will likely see some improvement in only one month with oral tranexamic acid, but best results may not be seen until three to four months of use. Tranexamic acid is also available in skin lightening creams and may be very effective topically.

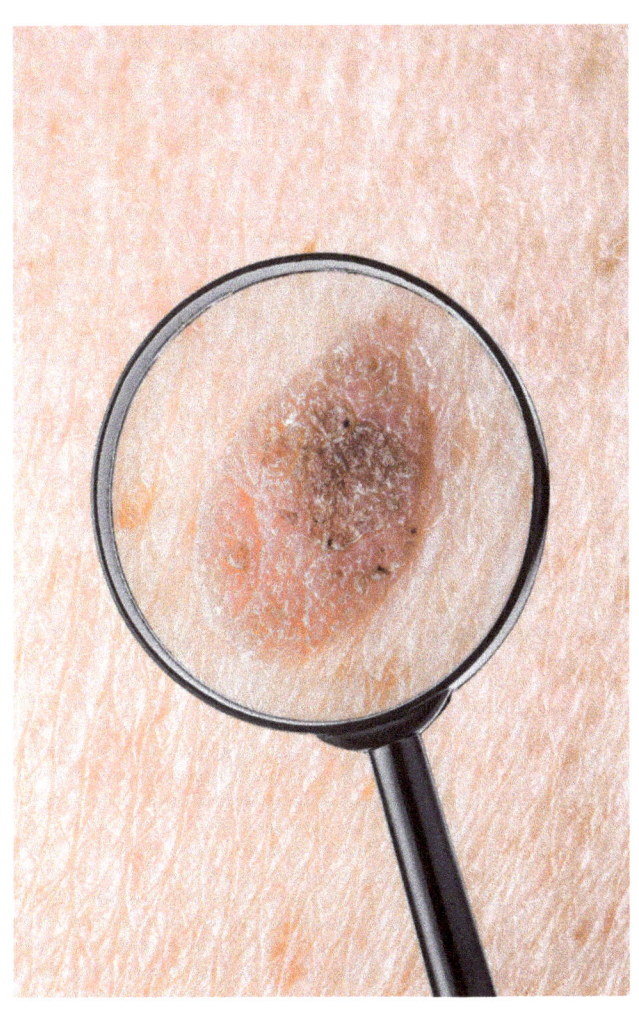

Brown and Red Blotchy Face, Neck, and Chest (Melasma, Poikiloderma)

When the brown spots on your face, neck, or chest are speckled and very stubborn, it could be melasma. If you have a combination of red and brown blotchy discoloration and dilated vessels on the neck and upper chest and sides of face, this could be Poikiloderma. Both melasma and Poikiloderma have a combination of brown discoloration and vascular changes in the skin that can give red blotchy discoloration, too. They are both worsened by sun, light, heat, and hormone changes. They can be seen in women and men. If you suffer from these problems, they can be improved and sometimes, quickly in a month or less, but it is crucial that you avoid sun, heat, and hormone irregularities to maintain your good results. No frequenting saunas, hot showers, or hot tubs. While there is no perfect cure for melasma or Poikiloderma yet, there are lots of remedies that help.

Topical retinoids, hydroquinone, and tranexamic acid creams are helpful for both melasma and Poikiloderma as are products containing kojic acid, licorice root extract, and niacinamide. For faster improvement, a light and/or laser treatment at the dermatologist's office would be best. Intense-pulsed or broad-band light and pulsed-dye laser are helpful for Poikiloderma as well as laser and energy device treatments that stimulate skin collagen and elastin formation and skin tightening. There is still no perfect laser treatment for melasma. In fact, many laser treatments worsen melasma, but some of the tattoo removal lasers, when done gently, can be helpful.

Benign Seborrheic Keratosis

If you have a brown spot on your skin that is changing in color or size rapidly within three months that may be suspicious and you should seek help from your dermatologist. There are common wart-like growths, which seem to change on adult skin called seborrheic keratoses. These skin growths are always changing in color, texture, and size and, despite their changes, are completely benign. Unfortunately, we all get these, sometimes very unattractive growths called keratoses with age and they get confused with moles and skin cancers all the time, even by some doctors. Most dermatologists know how to spot these sneaky keratoses by their wart-like, sandpaper texture. They are more like barnacles on our skin than true moles. They can be improved at home with moisturizers and some home wart remedies. See chapter 8 (Anti-aging) for further tips on treating these.

Finally, whether you have a prescription or not, when you are battling brown spots on the skin, as I mentioned earlier when discussing melasma, it is crucial that you avoid sun, heat, and the common chemical sunscreens.

All of these can worsen your brown spot condition quickly. Even saunas, hot tubs, and hot workouts. Even sun through most windows is harmful unless you can confirm the window contains a broad-spectrum UV block. If your car windows do not have adequate sun protection, it is possible to install a UV protective film at a car tint place. To see which UV film brands are best, try going to the Skin Cancer Foundation website and search for UV car tint or films under recommended sun protection products.

How Best to Protect from the Sun?

I recommend that if you are going to be outside for more than ten minutes, then you should apply sunblock, minimum SPF 30, to your skin. It is best to choose a mineral sunblock for your face, rather than chemical sunscreens. Mineral sunblocks have the following key ingredients: titanium dioxide and/or zinc oxide. Both these ingredients in sunblocks work by repelling sunrays off your skin. Chemical sunscreens like avobenzone / Parsol 1789, cinnamic aldehyde, oxybenzone, octinoxate, and octisalate absorb the sunrays hitting your skin and convert them to heat. This is problematic as it may heat, inflame, or irritate the skin, causing irritant rashes, or worsen brown discoloration or melasma. Chemical sunscreens have been found to appear in your blood stream within an hour of application, and we do not know if that is safe. In addition, some chemical sunscreens, oxybenzone, and octinoxate have been reported to damage the environment. Hawaii and Key West banned those chemical sunscreens in an effort to protect coral reefs.

Unfortunately, chemical sunscreens are still rampant on the skin care and makeup market and are often mixed in moisturizers and makeup. When someone is sensitive to sunscreen or gets a rash on their skin after application, it is most likely due to the chemical screens; either causing irritation or allergy. Less commonly, some people are sensitive to sun from a disease or medication they take. Women on birth control or hormone supplements will be more sensitive to sun and should be extra cautious to avoid, or they may get not only burns but unattractive brown spots and melasma. Some high blood pressure medications and antibiotics can make us very sensitive to the sun.

I cannot say enough about the importance of not trusting sunblock alone to provide full UV protection and it should be combined with use of wide-brimmed hats, long sleeves, and shade. I have seen many people who swear to me that they have used sunblock and they come into my office fried, as red as a tomato. Sunscreens and sunblocks may degrade with heat and time stored in your car or house and they are difficult to apply evenly and thoroughly. Many sunblock manufacturers have elegant face mineral sunblocks that are tinted with a light makeup so they do not look as pasty white. I recommend these tinted blocks for both men and women. They are natural appearing. They do not clog pores and do not usually look like visible makeup.

For more on sunblocks, go to the skin cancer foundation website: www.skincancer.org.

.

Chapter 4

Fix the Scars Quickly

Body Wounds on the Skin

A few words on skin wounds and healing them as quickly as possible. A good rule of thumb when it comes to how fast a wound will heal is: the further the skin from the heart or the further from good circulation, the more slowly that wound will heal. For example, a leg wound tends to heal slower than a shoulder or arm wound. In addition, the pinker and more vascular the skin, the faster the healing. Scalp and face wounds tend to heal the fastest, as they have a very rich blood supply. To speed healing of a skin scrape, scratch, or wound, it is important that the wound has good circulation.

Compress and Elevate

If you have a leg wound and you also happen to have spider veins or varicose veins or a tendency to swell in your legs at the end of the day, then your leg wounds will struggle to heal even more. Spider and varicose veins and swelling in the legs are signs of poor circulation in the legs. Deoxygenated venous blood and all their waste pools in the varicose and spider veins giving them a bluish, greenish, or purple color, depending on their caliber. Doctors call this sluggish vein flow in our legs venous stasis. It can be seen in both men and women and tends to worsen with age. It can be inherited in the family. To improve the circulation and control this problem, whenever standing or sitting, you must wear compression support socks or hose of at least 20mmg hg pressure. Compression prevents buildup of the venous blood in the thinned varicose and spider veins but still allows entry of the new oxygenated blood in the thicker deeper arteries. It is pretty easy to find attractive and comfortable compression socks nowadays.

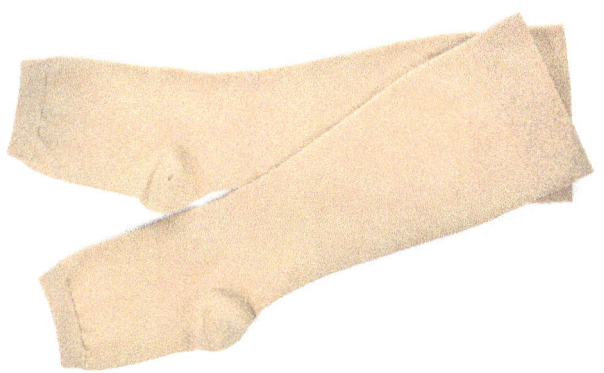

Typical Compression Socks. You Can Find Them in All Different Colors and Covering the Whole Foot.

My office staff and I wear them every day just to prevent ugly spider veins and aching or soreness. You can purchase good compression socks and hose at medical supply stores, sock stores, pharmacies, and on the internet.

When to Compress and Not to Compress

The circulation improves when sleeping or lying down or when the legs are elevated to chest level or higher and you may be able to remove your compression. While exercising, the muscles in the legs improve circulation and you may be able to remove the compression. If you have a forearm or hand wound, it may help to wrap a compression bandage and elevate the arm or hand with a sling. This will reduce fluid buildup, swelling, bruising, and speed healing.

Another few words on improving circulation near the skin wound. With a fresh wound there may be natural swelling and inflammation, which is your body doing everything it is supposed to do to help the wound heal.

This is all helpful to the skin but too much swelling after the first few days can start to interfere with healing. That's when compression and elevation become more important for the extremities. Usually it is not recommended to do heat pads to a fresh skin wound. Gentle or mild heat may be suitable for a distal extremity skin wound like on the toe or foot where you believe the skin temperature is below normal. A too cold foot or toe may also delay healing. Note, this is very different from when you have a fresh muscle or bony wound in your body where ice packs and elevation may be advised to control inflammation.

As you can see there is a delicate balance to healing your skin well and you can over or underdo it.

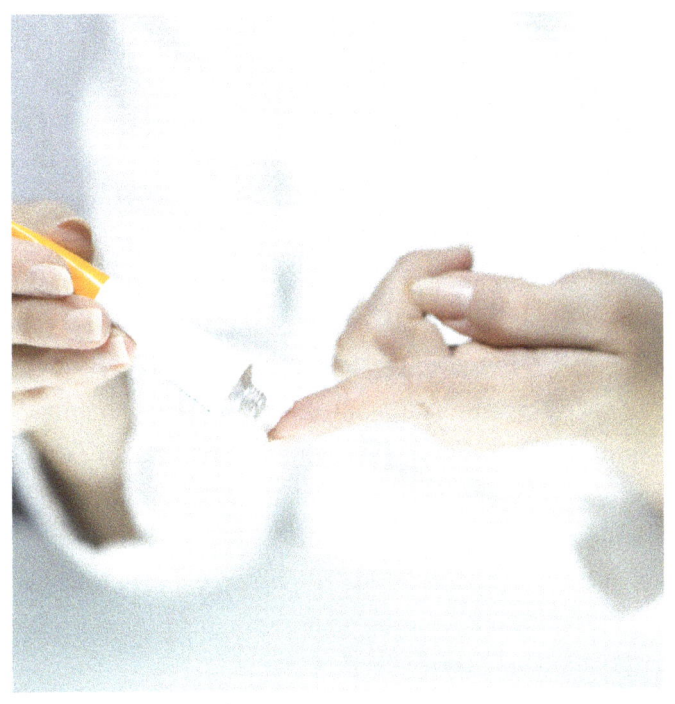

Wound Gels, Ointments, and Patches

As far as what you should apply on your wound to help it heal. For many years, dermatologists and other wound management doctors would recommend applying antibiotic ointment for five days. That has changed in the last decade since numerous studies showed that it is not necessary and tends to cause problems with allergy or sensitivity. Instead, it was found that moisture is necessary for fast wound healing but can be in the form of white Petrolatum (Vaseline or Aquaphor or similar) and does not need to be an antibiotic. I recommend applying this bland ointment to your wound two to three times a day or enough, so the wound does not dry out for at least five days.

If the wound is on the face, then five days or less of ointment application should not give acne. By one week, most wounds are no longer raw and you can switch from applying an ointment to a white cream or moisturizing cream. Many people give up their wound care too early and stop after the ointment stage and then wonder why their wound looks so discolored, dry, and is so itchy. Keep moisturizing the wound daily with a moisturizing cream for a complete month and avoid sun to it and it should keep improving. Sometimes, even with all the correct measures, a wound may not be done healing for many months. For discolored wounds that are no longer raw, you can try home treatment with serums or lotions that contain the following brown fading ingredients: tranexamic acid, azelaic acid, hydroquinone, licorice root, vitamin C, kojic acid, and niacinamide. Persistent discoloration or texture problems can often be helped with light or laser treatments at the dermatologist's office.

When a Wound May Scar

If you are concerned that your wound is scarring or going to scar and you want to know what is best to apply. First, it is important to calm any inflammation that is still present and may increase the risk of scarring. See Chapter 2 if you forget how to do that. The following steps are equally important: apply moisturizer twice daily and avoid the sun. Do not squeeze, pick, or pull off a scab.

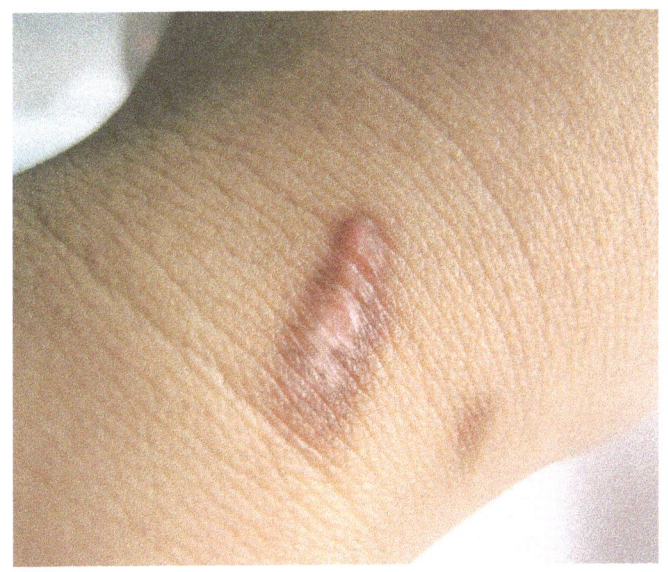

After one week of ointment application to your fresh skin wound, you can apply a fragrance-free moisturizing cream. You may switch from ointment to cream at about one week. Once a wound is no longer raw, usually a week or less after the injury, you may start applying a scar treatment product before your moisturizing cream.

Currently on the market, the best home scar treatment products for scars that are raised/thickened contain silicone. It can be applied as a cream or adhesive patch. Either way, you may need to use the product for many months for full improvement, if the scar has already thickened. The onion bulb extract scar treatment gels or creams may be helpful for any kind of scar whether flat or raised but are not usually as powerful as the silicone products for raised scars. If you get a scar patch treatment, then you can still apply a moisturizer cream to the wound first and then finish with the patch. The patch may stay in place for many days according to package instructions. If it's a scar gel or cream, then apply that first before a moisturizer as you would not want anything blocking penetration to remedy the scar.

Laser and light treatments for scars can be very helpful. The laser treatments may include injected medications and need to be repeated multiple times over a few months. If you have thirty days and can get into the dermatologist, sometimes one light or laser treatment will still be helpful and heal by thirty days. It is possible that by combining this first laser or light treatment with all the home remedies I discussed above, you will get great results in just thirty days.

Keloids and Hypertrophic Scars

Technically, keloids are tumor-like scars where their size grows beyond the original scar edges. A scar that is just simply raised or thicker but still within the margins of the original wound is simply a 'hypertrophic scar.' Keloids and hypertrophic scars are treated similarly but keloids tend to be more stubborn and less responsive. I have already discussed some of the treatments for these scars above but will elaborate here.

At home, one may treat a keloid or hypertrophic scar with silicone-based scar remedies and compression. For keloids on the earlobes, there are pressure earrings that can be purchased and worn for months as treatment. The compression can be very effective for shrinking the keloid or preventing growth of a new keloid. It is best to do both; the silicone-based scar cream or tape and compression together for established keloids and continue the treatment daily for many months or until improvement is seen.

At the dermatologist's office, hypertrophic scars and keloids can be treated with a combination of steroid injections, fluorouracil injections, and laser and light treatments. These treatments often need to be repeated two to five times depending on the size and location of the scar. While we do not have a perfect cure for scars nowadays, we do have remedies that can improve the scars significantly and sometimes come close to perfection.

Chapter 5

Stop the Eczema, Rashes, and Dry Skin

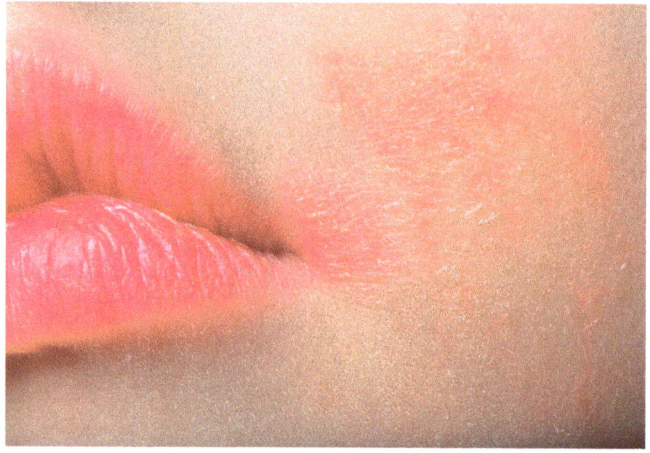

Irritant Eczema

It is common to confuse infections, pre-cancers, and even skin cancers with a rash or vice versa. Ok, that was confusing, wasn't it? As a dermatologist, I see this confusion about our skin every day. Someone will come in with an obvious pre-cancer or skin cancer spot on their face when they had been treating it with an eczema cream. Other times, I have seen people come in with dandruff on their face and they were treating it with an eczema or acne treatment, which may just make it worse. Dandruff is essentially an inflammatory and oily yeast infection, called seborrheic dermatitis by dermatologists. It not only occurs on the scalp but can be on the face and chest.

Knowing what you think may be an eczema or a rash, may not actually be that, as I demonstrated above. You need to take care in how long you try a home treatment without getting professional help. In most cases, you can try common sense home treatments for your rash for at least a couple weeks before deciding you need further expert help.

Here is my disclaimer to trying remedies at home. If your symptoms are severe with severe itch or discomfort, then it may not be reasonable to keep trying things at home. It is probably time to call the doctor. Or if your problem persists past thirty days despite your best home efforts, then it may also be time to call the doctor. In recent years, many dermatologists offer telemedicine where you can send a photo of your rash or skin spot to them via text or e-mail and you can get a diagnosis and starting place. See if that is an option with your doctor, if you are having trouble going in person.

Correcting the pH

An important step to controlling face rashes of all kinds, even acne, is to correct the pH of your skin. Normal skin pH is about 5.5. When your skin pH is off, even by a little, you are more likely to have a skin problem.

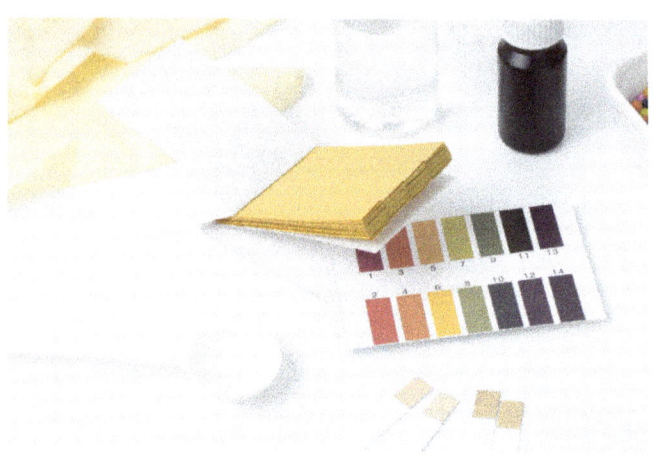

Studies have shown that people with rashes or acne tend to have more alkaline skin pH and need to lower or acidify their skin to improve things. I do not recommend you test your skin pH which is neither convenient nor easy. It is enough to use an acidic cleanser or toner or leave on topical skin treatment that is designed to correct skin pH. These special pH-correcting skin products will usually say 'corrects skin pH' on the label.

I have met lots of people over the years that think they are being a hero by washing their face with simple water and no soap or cleanser. Tap water that you use to wash your face is usually alkaline, so it is not a good idea to wash your face with plain tap water and no cleanser. The cleanser you choose should be a gentle cleanser that is both acidic and contains healthy lipids (fats) to repair your skin barrier. I do not like to advertise name brands, which is why I am not listing options. If you note the key ingredients that I recommend, you should be able to find a good and safe cleanser. Look for a cleanser with the following ingredients:

pH-correcting, fragrance-free, healthy lipids (glycerin, ceramides.)

If you do very vigorous exercise with heating of your skin and sweat, you may increase the pH of your skin so it becomes vulnerable to rashes or acne. This is why it may be important to gently cleanse your face with an acidic pH correcting cleanser after your workout. If you do mild to moderate exercise, you are less likely to affect your skin pH.

If you are prone to eczema, it is important you understand what we know about the causes and triggers of eczema in order to quickly get it under control. I will spend some time here going over what you should know about your eczema. Dermatologists have studied eczema for many decades now and have figured out more and more about what causes it. People who have eczema tend to also have asthma, hay fever, seasonal allergies as well, or that stuff will run in the family. When you have eczema there is usually a problem with the barrier or protective function of your skin, where the skin cell barrier does not form properly each month. Often there is not enough natural fat or lipids in the skin. When the skin barrier is weak, it will let in more things like allergies and infections. This is why we tend to see more skin allergies and infections in people with eczema.

Fixing the Skin Barrier

When you have eczema or dry skin, it is crucial that you repair the skin barrier by adding what is missing and using a moisturizing cream fortified with ceramides every day for twice a day. A good time to apply the moisturizer is after a bath or shower and repeat twelve hours later. Note that I said a 'cream' and not a lotion. Lotions, unless they have ceramides and are designed for eczema, tend to be lighter and less moisturizing than creams.

When choosing skin creams for dry or eczema-prone skin, always avoid fragrances and dyes. Look for the following ingredients: ceramides, omega fatty acids, evening primrose oil, sunflower seed oil, linoleic acid, dimethicone, niacinamide, mineral oil, glycerin, urea, chamomile, and aloe vera.

To maintain a healthy skin barrier, avoid excessive washing and wetting of the skin. If you do housework like dishes, always wear protective gloves. Dish detergents along with frequent wetting in alkaline tap water is very irritating to the skin. Avoid long hot baths, showers, and hot tubs if you tend to have dry, irritated, or itchy skin.

Fixing Your Skin Flora Balance

A major trigger of eczema and rashes is having your normal bacteria and yeast or flora getting unbalanced. This can happen with under-washing, over-washing, oral or topical antibiotics, hormone changes, stress, and possible dietary changes. While the many causes of unbalanced skin flora may seem overwhelming, you can try to focus on how to fix the imbalance.

It has been shown that right before a flare-up of eczema or new rash the skin flora tends to be imbalanced, where there is less healthy mixed flora. Your normal

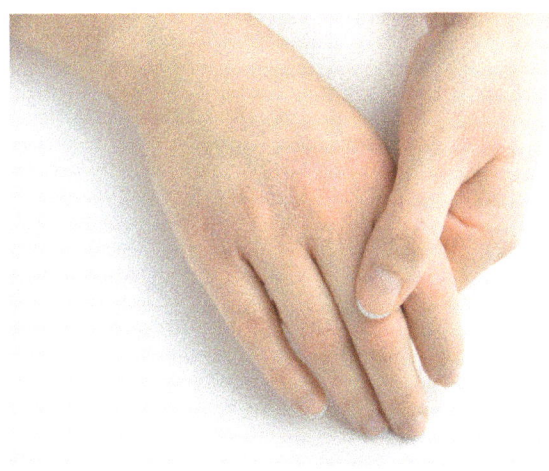

skin flora can rebalance with all of the following steps: proper gentle daily skin cleansing, stopping topical or oral antibiotics, daily moisturizing, healthy diet, balanced hormones, and skin pH-balancing serums or gels or sprays. The latter option, skin pH-balancing products have become more common and more available in the marketplace in recent years. They can be found in the store with 'pH correcting' on their labels. These products help gently acidify your skin to a normal skin pH, which encourages a healthier mix of skin flora. Some of these products are from thermal springs in Europe where the water is enriched with healthy bacteria and anti-inflammatory elements like selenium and strontium.

Sensitive Skin

If you think you have sensitive skin and your skin seems to react easily to products, you are probably wondering if all of these recommendations I offer apply to you. The answer is *yes*. This book applies to you too. I wrote this section to highlight the key skin care concepts you need to keep in mind when caring for sensitive skin.

Cosmeceuticals are skin products that have function that lies somewhere in between a cosmetic and a medicine grade product. Incorporating cosmeceuticals into your daily skin care regimen when you have sensitive skin should be done with caution. Many herbal ingredients are irritants or allergens to sensitive skin. It is wise to start with products that do not contain many ingredients and must be tested on a small are of your skin first, such as the inside of your wrist or the side of your face by the ear. Test for a few days before applying to a larger area of your skin.

I get asked all the time which skin care line is best for sensitive skin. The truth is there are many brands that are great for sensitive skin and I do not want to plug any particular one. I recommend you read the labels carefully and select those that say things like: fragrance-free, dye-free, hypoallergenic, non-comedogenic, paraben-free, PEG, and formaldehyde-free. If these products still cause irritation or rash, then a bland ointment may be the only safe option like: white petrolatum, True Lipids ointment, Vaseline, or Aquaphor ointment. These thicker ointments are fine to apply daily for moisturizing the body. Ointments are the most moisturizing and are not recommended on oily skin areas for more than a few days or acne may occur.

Cleansing is still important when you have sensitive skin. You should gently cleanse your face before applying your lotion or creams or makeup. Cleanse gently with fingertips lathering a liquid cleanser and avoid using wash cloths or rotating brushes. There are many gentle face and body cleansers available that work for this purpose. Okay, I will give a brand name suggestion here, but I have no interest or relation to the manufacturer of this product. Cetaphil cleanser is one of the most studied and trusted by dermatologists for sensitive skin.

With sensitive skin, try using creams rather than lotions as creams tend to be less irritating. Avoid gels which are the most drying unless you follow it immediately with a soothing cream. Serums have become popular in recent years and they tend to be liquid or oily. They are often tolerated well by all skin types, depending on their active ingredients. Some people experience acne flare-ups with vitamin C serums.

With sensitive skin, it is best to use only mineral makeups and physical sunblocks rather than chemical makeups and sunscreens. Never cleanse your face more than twice a day, if you are sensitive. When choosing skin products to help rejuvenate sensitive skin, consider alternative ingredients to the potentially irritating retinoids and acid peels, such as the following examples: stem cell growth factor cream (SkinMedica TNS, NeoCutis), antioxidant-rich cream (Skinceuticals), peptides (Regenerist). Once again, I have no personal interest in these brands, which are examples of a growing market of rejuvenating growth factor skin creams.

Sweaty Skin and Heat Rashes

Rashes from sweat and heat tend to occur in areas of friction and our skin folds: groin, armpits, under breasts, and belly folds. Such heat rashes can sometimes be prevented by keeping your skin folds cool and dry. Heat and sweat rashes are seen more often in athletes that are not keeping cool and dry, overweight people that are not staying fit, and with diseases like uncontrolled diabetes and hyperhidrosis (excessive sweating). Start by wearing more breathable clothing. You can apply a thin layer of antiperspirant to sweat-prone areas, even if they are not armpits. You can also apply powders that dry the area or barrier creams that contain zinc oxide. Friction rashes can be seen in some athletes. For example, bikers tend to get groin rashes from the friction, heat, sweat, and occlusion to their bottoms. We also see friction rashes in the folds of people who are overweight. If you already have the rash and failed the prevention step, then keep reading for tips on how to control it.

Start by treating the friction or heat rash with a hydrocortisone cream. Hydrocortisone 2% creams are available without a prescription at most pharmacies. If you have itching or soreness or scattered pustules or pimple-like bumps at the edge, there may be a yeast infection. You can treat that with an anti-yeast cream like Lotrimin, which can also be found easily in most pharmacies.

Sometimes sweating is so severe that antiperspirant seems not enough. Be sure that you tried a 'clinical strength' antiperspirant like aluminum chloride 20% before concluding it's not enough. If you have tried the strong antiperspirants, then it is best to get further evaluated with a dermatologist to see whether the sweat is primary or secondary 'hyperhidrosis' and then prescription treatments can be discussed. Primary hyperhidrosis is excessive sweating that is inherited or running in the family.

Secondary hyperhidrosis is excessive sweating caused by something else, like a disease or a medication.

Occasionally, less common rashes like psoriasis will occur in the folds of the skin. So, if your rash seems stubborn and not responding to the tactics mentioned earlier, then it may be time to have a dermatologist look at it and rule out possibilities like an infection or psoriasis. I have seen people complain about a bumpy heat rash, and when I look, I see pimple-like bumps centered around the pores and scattered all over the body. This is called folliculitis and typically goes away with the following anti-yeast or anti-microbial remedies: dandruff shampoos that contain the active ingredient zinc pyrithione, chlorhexidine (Hibiclens) liquid antiseptic soap, or oral anti-yeast or oral antibiotic pills that are prescribed.

Dry Bump on the Arms

One of the most common questions I get asked as a dermatologist is, "What are these bumps on my arms and how do I get rid of them?"

In many people, these bumps will not only be on arms but also on the thighs, low back, butt, and face. Sometimes the bumps are skin-toned, other times pink. They tend to have a rough, sandpaper-like texture. When on the arms and shoulders, they can resemble acne. Dermatologists call this bumpy dry skin condition 'keratosis pilaris.' It is believed that four out of ten people have this benign condition. Most dermatologists think of it as a subtype of mild eczema. It can be treated and controlled, but not cured. The most common way to treat it is with an exfoliating moisturizer cream. Many of these creams contain mild fruit acids. A popular and less expensive acid cream that is effective is 'lactic acid cream.' Test the cream in a small area before going big, just in case you get stinging or irritation. Exfoliating creams like these will cause your dead skin cells to shed faster and may make your skin more sensitive to sun and burn more easily. Always remember to protect from the sun when you are using such creams.

Cracked and Peeling Feet

Persistent cracked, peeling feet may not be just dry skin. Sometimes the dry and peeling feet can be eczema, psoriasis, or a fungal infection. These problems will usually have symptoms of itch or pain but, sometimes, need to be diagnosed by the dermatologist. Other times, it is just dry skin which is worsened by friction, barefoot activities, or genetics. Dry and cracked feet can run in some families. The dry areas on the feet may look yellow like a callus. Dermatologists call this problem 'keratoderma' as it involves thickened keratin.

If there is a lot of peeling, then an exfoliating moisturizer or gentle chemical peel product may be helpful. Application with a home microdermabrasion device can help the lotion better penetrate the thick peeling layers. After the exfoliating step, then it is necessary to apply a moisturizing cream at least once a day and twice a day, when flaring up.

When the dry, peeling feet runs in the family, unfortunately, there is no cure at this time and just ways to manage the problem. You will need to find an exfoliating and moisturizing routine that works for you and that you can do a few times a week as needed for maintenance.

Dry and Peeling Lips

Some people struggle with dry lips more than others. Lips tend to get drier and peel in dry climates and in people or kids, who lick their lips too much. Saliva can be very irritating to the outside of the lips. Sometimes your lips can peel repeatedly from sun damage and pre-cancer changes. Sun damaged lips are seen more often in adults and elderly. Sun damage causing pre-cancer change usually looks like circular scaly pink spots around or on the lips that won't heal. If you suspect you have this, it is time to visit the dermatologist.

Lip Sugar Scrubs

Avoiding licking and apply a moisturizing lip balm to your lips after every meal and again at bedtime, which should help improve the dryness. Gentle exfoliation with a lip sugar scrub is helpful. Apply the gritty sugar scrub with your fingertips in a circular motion and then wipe off the excess and grit with a damp soft towel. Then, finish by applying a moisturizer lip balm. You can repeat these steps with the sugar scrub followed by lip balm daily, as needed. Mineral oil, beeswax, shea butter, jojoba oil, and coconut oil are some moisturizing ingredients you should look for in your moisturizing lip balms.

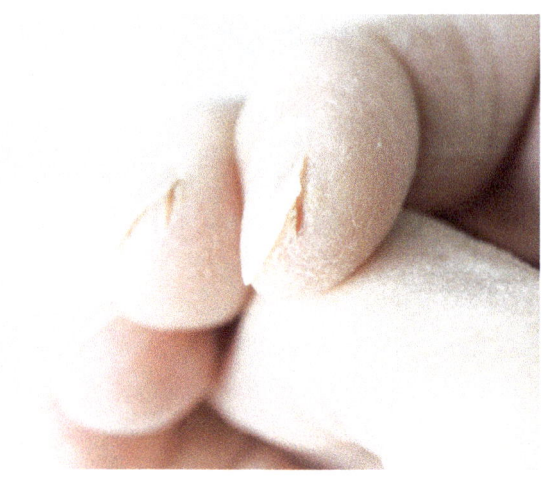

Dry, fissured fingertips

Dry and Peeling Fingertips

Peeling, cracked, and even painful fingertips is a common dry skin problem of the hands. It is seen more often in people who wash or wet their hands excessively.

The first step to controlling the dry fingertips is to avoid excessive wetting and washing. Try to wear protective gloves while doing work that involves wetting your hands like doing dishes, cleaning, cooking, and hairstyling etc. Then, apply a healing ointment like Vaseline or Aquaphor or CeraVe and massage it into your fingertips three to four times daily until healed. If a crack is very painful, then you may want to put an antibiotic ointment on it three times daily for a few days and treat for a possible infection. If this does not work and it is still sore, you may have a yeast, fungal or even herpes infection of the finger. Bacterial or herpes infections of the fingers tend to be more painful, red, and swollen. A yeast infection of the finger is typically pink, sore, but less angry-looking, and usually resolves with clotrimazole cream. When herpes infects the finger, it's like getting a cold sore on the finger. This can be pretty painful. Some finger infections can get pretty serious quickly so when in doubt, just see your doctor to figure it out.

To prevent recurrence of dry, peeling, and cracked fingertips, I recommend a hand barrier cream. These can be found among other hand creams at the store and will usually have the word 'barrier' on the label. The active moisturizing barrier ingredient in these creams is usually a silicone derivative. These barrier creams help protect your hands from water and can even repel water.

Nail Infections

We discussed some common infections of the finger earlier, but now we will review some nail infections. Sometimes staph, strep, or other bacteria can infect the skin around or underneath the nail. Usually there will be pain, redness, swelling, and pus or drainage. A green, discolored nail can be seen with pseudomonas bacterial infection. For a green nail, you may be able to cure it with home vinegar soaks. You can add a tablespoon of white vinegar to a pint or two cups of water, and soak for five minutes three times a day. Just dip your toe in the dilute vinegar. For further help and to verify what kind of nail infection you may have, it is best to see the dermatologist.

A more common nail infection, especially in women or men who get manicures or pedicures regularly, are yeast and fungal infections of the nails. Both yeast and fungus nail infections can be tender. We all have yeast and fungus on our skin as part of our normal skin flora and sometimes the trauma of a manicure or pedicure will introduce the flora under our nail. Aggressive nail treatments should be avoided. Ask your nail technician to be gentler and not trim, dig, or push at cuticles too much. Check that your manicurist sterilizes all instruments and that files and buffs are not used on anyone else before you. It is easy to spread these infections by contact. I have also seen warts spread in this way after a pedicure or manicure with a second-hand file or buff. Just as with the finger as I explained earlier, a clue to telling a bacterial infection of the nail is that such infections tend to drain pus and are brighter red and more swollen. The yeast or fungal infections can linger longer for weeks or months and be more indolent. Dermatologists call a chronic or longer lasting yeast infection of the nail 'paronychia.'

If you are concerned that you are getting a yeast or fungal infection after a nail treatment, there is no harm in applying a few doses of a topical anti-yeast/anti-fungal. Clotrimazole or miconazole antifungals are available without a prescription in the foot aisle of most pharmacies. Tea tree oil nail treatments sometimes work for this, too. I recommend applying it two to three times a day for a few days until your symptoms subside. If your fungal nail infection is longer established, then sometimes these over-the-counter remedies will still work with persistence and use for a few weeks. If not, then it is time to see your dermatologist for a prescription.

Things That Look Like Eczema but Aren't

If you are sure that you have eczema, which tends to look like red scaly patches that have blurred borders, then it is best to try and calm the inflammation as soon as possible. First, eliminate all skin products that contain fragrance or dyes and stick with only very bland and sensitive skin products. Gently clean your skin daily but take care to avoid over-washing and over-wetting. People who have jobs that involve wetting or washing their hands a lot tend to get hand eczema. Be sure and read the 'calm and stop the inflammation' Chapter 2 carefully to help calm your eczema. Read on for common skin problems that can pretend to be eczema.

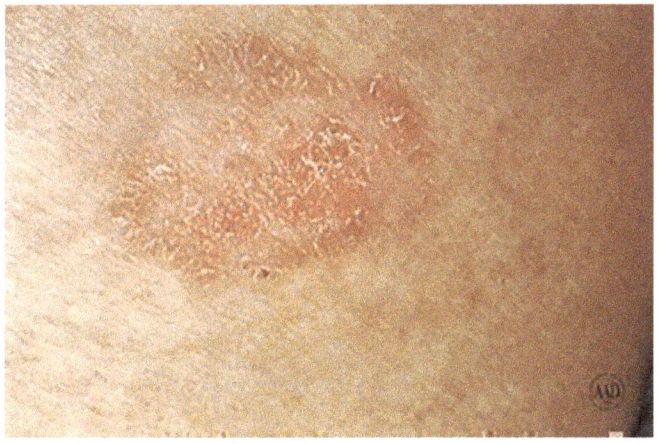

Squamous Cell Carcinoma Shown Above. Note the Confusing Eczema-Like Appearance.

If you have a circular, rashy, and eczema-like spot on your skin and it keeps coming back despite trying a topical steroid cream, then you may have a growth and not a dermatitis. Such growths may be pre-cancer or skin cancer and should be checked by a dermatologist as soon as possible. Eczema is usually not as stubborn as a pre-cancer or skin cancer and will resolve or improve easily with a topical steroid.

If your face seems to be breaking out with pimples but there also seems to be a rash at the same time, you may have a non-eczema rash like perioral dermatitis, rosacea, yeast acne, or seborrheic dermatitis (dandruff). These are best distinguished with the help of a dermatologist.

Things That Look Like Acne but Aren't

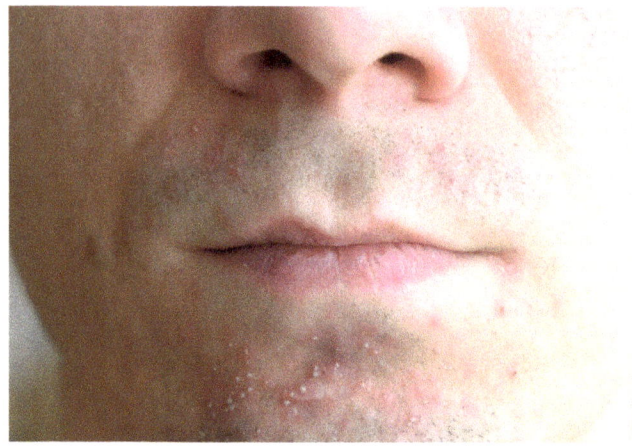

Perioral dermatitis

There are a lot of rashes that mimic acne such as rosacea, perioral/peri nasal dermatitis, dandruff, and fungal or yeast infections. Basically, all of these can have pustules and inflamed skin bumps. It can get tricky, even for some doctors to sort them out. Other than getting the story behind your rash, one of the ways we figure out which bump is which is by looking closer at the size and locations of the pustules and bumps on your skin. I will give some common examples now to illustrate this.

If you have bumps in the T-zone of the face; forehead, nose, chin, and medial cheeks, you are likely to have acne or dandruff (seborrheic dermatitis). If these bumps are mixed in with blackheads and whiteheads, then it is likely you have acne. If you have bumps on the nose and cheeks with swollen capillaries or veins and easy flushing, then you may have rosacea. If you have bumps coalescing to a rash and concentrated around your mouth and nose, and sometimes the eyes, then you may have perioral/peri nasal dermatitis.

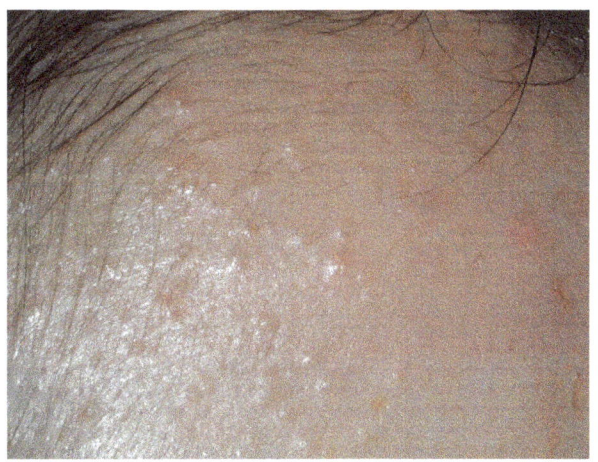

Pityrosporum yeast acne. Note how it looks just like regular acne, but smaller, rash-like, and involving the hair-line.

If the bumps are small and located on the forehead, hairline, upper chest and back and you also have oily skin and oily scalp, then you may have yeast, acne, or pityrosporum acne/folliculitis. I realize this all seems too simple to be true but these are just the common and typical presentations.

If you want to more firmly diagnose yourself with yeast acne, there is a simple trick I like to do in the office that you can try at home. If you happen to have a black light or Wood's lamp at home. Those are the lights that can be used to find dog or cat urine around your house. They are not black Halloween light bulbs. The bulbs actually look purple. They sell them cheap at pet stores and on the internet. You will need to sit in a dark room with a family member or friend or a mirror to assist you with the light. Turn off the lights, close window shades, and, preferably, go into a windowless room and shine the black light on your skin. If you see lots of coral pink colored tiny bumps that look like pink glitter, it is the pityrosporum (also known as Malassezia) yeast. A little of it scattered on our skin is normal but if you see a lot of the pink glitter clustering by your acne, then you probably have yeast acne. To treat this kind of acne, I recommend an extra strength dandruff shampoo with the active ingredient zinc pyrithione to the area. Let it sit for five minutes before rinsing and repeat daily for a couple weeks, as needed. If that doesn't work, you can get a prescription from your dermatologist.

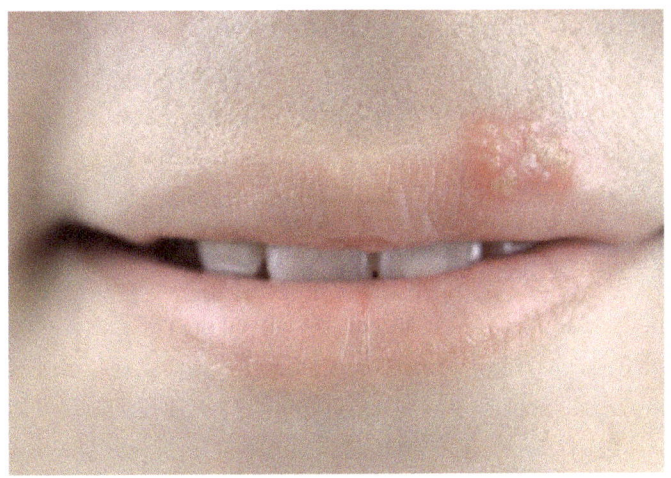
Herpes simplex infection (cold sore)

Urgent Infections That Can Mimic Acne or Eczema

Herpes cold sores typically begin as a tingling and sore spot. These sores can be anywhere on the skin but more commonly found on the lip and nose. The sore usually starts with a sting or tingle. It shows up in the same place on your skin each time and evolves to a swollen pink pustule or blister and then scabs over. If left untreated, it may take a couple weeks to heal. Herpes simplex virus comes in many strains and may show up not only on the face, fingers, buttocks, shoulder, back, buttocks, sides, and genitals. It is transmitted by contact and can be passed sexually. Impetigo and recurrent staph or strep skin infections can look similar to a herpes cold sore but the clue to differentiating the two is that bacterial skin infections with staph or strep do not usually recur in the exact same area on the skin the way herpes does. Another clue to a herpes infection is they irritate your nerves, giving a tingle, burn, or itch.

The first step to healing a cold sore quickly is to find an antiviral medication. There are antiviral creams available without a prescription like penciclovir, Denavir, etc. Oral lysine supplements have never been consistently shown to clear herpes infections. If you still believe in the power of Lysine, they are usually safe if taken no more than twice daily. All of these treatments discussed are for sale at most pharmacies. Your doctor can prescribe a prescription oral antiviral like acyclovir, valacyclovir, or famciclovir. The key is to start treatment as soon as possible and the sore will go away faster. Sometimes herpes cold sores get infected with bacteria too, so it is a good idea to apply an antibiotic ointment to prevent this secondary infection while the cold sore is healing. Also, moisture heals wounds faster, so applying an ointment should speed healing as well.

If you get cold sores five or more times per year, then you may want to consider getting a prescription oral antiviral medication to take as chronic prophylaxis.

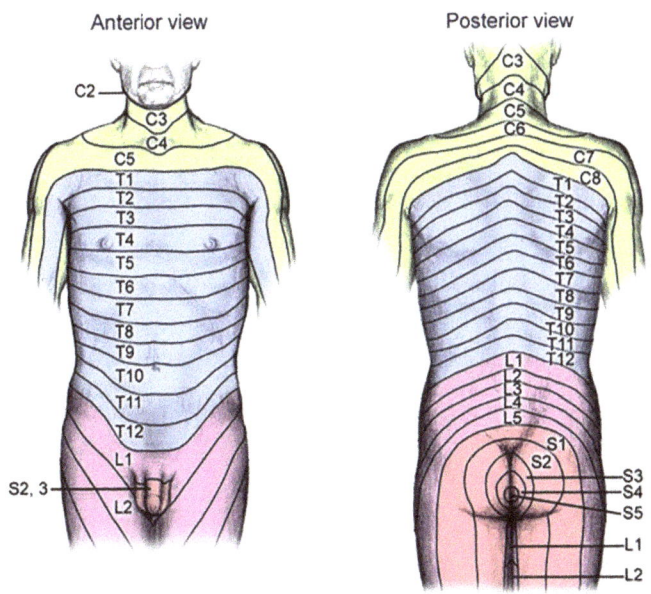

Dermatomes of the skin are shown here. Shingles occurs along one or a few dermatomes.

Cold sores are triggered by stress, sun, and irritation on the skin. Herpes simplex and shingles get confused a lot, so I will try to clear up the differences so that you can spot them earlier. Shingles, especially, is best caught early to prevent complications.

Shingles and How It Is Different Than Herpes

Shingles is caused by a different virus than herpes, which is known as the varicella zoster virus. This is the same virus that causes chicken pox, so anyone who has had chicken pox will have this virus hanging out dormant in their nervous system for lifelong. Under stress, the virus will come out along one to a few sensory nerves at a time and present as a blistering painful rash along the skin that is innervated by those nerves. A dermatome is an area on the skin that is innervated by a certain sensory nerve. You can look at a dermatome map and confirm which nerves are involved in your shingles infection. Shingles is considered a skin emergency because if not treated promptly, it can rarely result in prolonged awful nerve pain called 'post-herpetic neuralgia.' If you think you may have shingles, see a doctor as soon as possible. Adults and kids can get shingles. Some people, and even some doctors, confuse shingles with herpes and vice versa. Some of the confusion stems from the fact that both are painful and blistering. Shingles tends to run along a band-like dermatome of the skin whereas herpes will be in a smaller spot or cluster.

Shingles is contagious to others who have never been exposed to chicken pox. The chicken pox vaccine is a weakened version of the live virus. Once you have had the chicken pox vaccine, the virus can reactivate later in life as shingles but this is rare. There is also a vaccine for shingles that is recommended for people over 65, who are at greater risk of contracting shingles. If you have had a bout with shingles, you will likely be immune to a recurrence for about four to five years. So, we all can get shingles repeatedly. Unfortunately, there is no vaccine widely available yet for herpes simplex infection.

Finally, don't be a know it all, who doesn't know it all. Seek help with the dermatologist if you are not seeing improvement within one to two weeks of self-diagnosis and starting your chosen skin care regimen.

Chapter 6

Hives, Bug Bites, and Urgent Itches

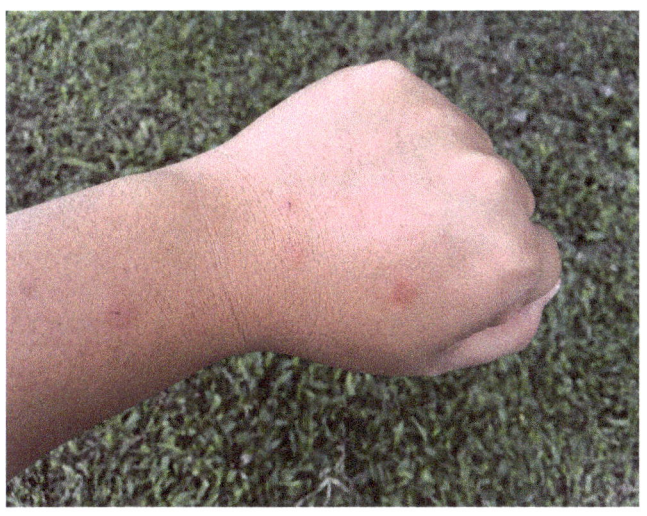

Mild hive bite reaction from insects. Note, central punctum and group of three bites.

In recent years, you can hear and read scary stories about travelers and bed bug infestations and mites. These are clean people with professional jobs that live in homes with white picket fences. We're not talking about homeless shelter situations. Bed bugs and mites need to be considered when you get itchy bumps that keep appearing over a few weeks to months after travel. Even if you are a CEO of a big corporation, some people will get hives as a reaction to bugs and insects and even, parasites.

First, let's review what hives and bug bites look like. Hives are itchy and red/white bumpy swellings on the skin. They tend to be white in the center with a red edge. They can occur in singles or clusters of many. Bug bites will usually have a central punctum or tiny hole with a hive around it. Sometimes, the bug or mite reaction can be just very small red bumpy swellings and not big swollen hives. The location of the bites on our skin is also a clue that you may have a bug infestation. Bugs prefer to bite wrists, ankles, hands, feet, and extremities over our core body. They prefer the cooler temperatures of our extremities. Bugs also like to bite in threes with three bumps near each other. Doctors like to call this phenomenon 'breakfast, lunch, and dinner.' It won't always be a cluster of exactly three but sometimes it is two or four bites. The point is that bugs rarely stop at one bite.

Don't think that just because your spouse or partner did not get the bug rash too, it's not bugs. Dermatologists see bug hypersensitivity (allergy) rashes affecting one partner and not the other, all the time. So, just because you're the only one with the rash in the family, it does not exclude the possibility of bugs. Some people can be bitten by bugs or mites but not get a significant reaction or rash. Other people always break out from bug or mite bites. See below for more discussion of allergy reactions to bug bites.

If you suspect you may have a bug or mite problem, the first step is to examine your clothes, bedding, bed, and luggage for possible culprits. Look on the internet for more images of pictures of bed bugs and mites, as well as cleaning tips. Never put suitcases on your bed, when packing and unpacking. I have seen people transfer bugs that way. The bugs can spread from a suitcase to a luggage rack or table too. Bugs love hiding inside and outside suitcases, wood frame furniture, or beds, mattress seams, and clothing, ugh!

While you are cleaning and debugging your home, luggage, and clothing, you can begin a treatment for your skin. The first-line remedy for mites (not bed bugs) on the skin is a prescription cream called 'permethrin.' You will need to see a physician to get this prescription. If it is other bugs, like bed bugs, then treatment of the skin rash may just require topical steroid creams, which can be prescribed by a doctor. Beware that after a rash caused by mites is treated with permethrin, some people may experience itching that persists for a month or more. This may be the hypersensitivity reaction. Taking an oral anti-histamine like loratadine can be helpful for itching from bug bites.

Allergy to Bug Bites

Some people are highly allergic or reactive to mosquito and other bug bites and will develop incredibly itchy hive-like bumps around their bug bites. If this sounds like you, then you can get relief with careful planning. Always carry bug repellant in high risk situations for bug bites. Picaridin is my preferred chemical bug repellant. The natural repellants may not work quite as well and DEET may be more toxic. Always wear long pants or put plenty of repellant on at night in a buggy place. I recommend even spraying your pant legs with the repellant. While in a buggy place, check your skin daily for bites so you can stay ahead of it and start appropriate treatment before your skin starts to react. Apply a topical steroid ointment or gel a few times a day to the bug bite to calm the inflammation and prevent it from escalating. If you know you get this overreaction to bug bites, then you may want to get a prescription topical steroid ointment from your doctor prior to travel or to keep at home. In addition to treating the bug bite hives with a topical steroid, you can take an oral antihistamine like loratadine. You may need to continue the treatment for a few days to heal the hives.

Sarna and Calamine lotions are not effective when you have this severe bite hive-like reaction. If your reaction is severe and hives seem to be spreading beyond your original bug bites, then you may need to go to an urgent care clinic for oral steroids. I know about bug bite allergy personally, as I suffer from this condition. It can be pretty embarrassing. The first time it happened when I was 25 with a date out to dinner and later that evening my legs were polka dotted with red swollen bumps. I tried Benadryl, cold bath, and Calamine and none of them was enough. I had to see the dermatologist urgently for steroids before I got relief from the insane itching. Now I know how to prevent this reaction following the steps I just taught you and it always works.

Plant Dermatitis (Poison Ivy)

Plant rashes or reactions typically show up the same day or within days of exposure to the plant, and tend to have a streak or scratched pattern. You may see lines or streaks of pink bumps or blisters. If you are concerned that you have a plant allergy rash or poison ivy, then the treatment is similar to the bug bite reaction treatments that I have described above. Begin with topical steroid ointments and oral antihistamines. If that is not adequate to control the itch or spread of this hypersensitivity rash, then you may need to go to an urgent care clinic or dermatologist for oral steroids. Poison ivy and similar plants (poison sumac and oak) spread by an oily resin from the plant. It can be on your clothes, skin, pets, and other belongings. Be sure to clean all that you could have come in contact with the resin. Some people, but not most, are very allergic to poison ivy and will get these insane reactions that require oral steroids to control.

Chapter 7

Quick Acne Fixes

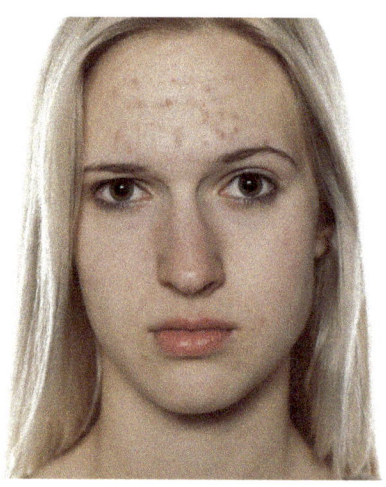

In this chapter I look forward to sharing with you some crucial steps to achieving clear skin. Let's begin by discussing the importance of a daily skin care routine. Unfortunately, there is no perfect lasting cure for acne yet. It would be nice if we could just apply a medicine once a week or once a month and keep the acne away, but I assure you that will not work. If you have acne and you want quick results and to sustain the results, you must commit to a daily routine that both prevents acne as well as treats the acne. Your dermatologist may prescribe you medications to take daily but it is not enough to use the medications. You must also avoid the triggers of acne on a daily basis. Think of it as an anti-acne lifestyle, just like if we want to stay fit and maintain our weight, we must diet and exercise. If you are reading this book to help your teenager with their acne or you are a teenager, you are probably getting concerned after hearing that a daily routine is needed. Many teens have trouble following the daily routine. This is usually because they are already very busy, and sometimes it is because they are not motivated to control their acne. If you think you have the motivation problem, then it is time to pause and consider the importance of having healthy skin for your social life, school, and work. The next thing you should pause to consider is that if you fail to control your acne well now, you may live to regret the permanent scars untreated acne will leave.

To help remember your daily routine, I recommend teens pair their acne-fighting steps with other necessary daily hygiene steps like teeth brushing or bathing. Keep your cleanser and acne medications visible on your bathroom counter near your other hygiene tools. Parent's may need to remind their teens and check in a couple times a week with reminders.

The routine is more than likely going to be as follows:
step 1 – cleanse
step 2 – tone
step 3 – apply medication

step 4 – moisturize or apply sunblock and/or makeup.

Acne Medications

In 2016 something exciting happened in the acne treatment world. The most important and most effective class of prescription topical acne medication, retinoids, went over-the-counter. Currently, the only available version of retinoid without prescription is adapalene gel (Differin gel). It is very effective for most mild to even moderate cases of facial acne. It is best used every night at bedtime, by applying a green pea size amount to the entire face. Results may not be visible for four to six weeks of use. Some people purge or worsen with a flare-up in the first couple weeks of application because it is so effective at surfacing deeper pimples. There is a prescription strength of adapalene gel available for more severe cases that your doctor can prescribe, as needed. All retinoids are sun-sensitizing where with continued use, you will burn more easily or be more vulnerable to sun damage. I will discuss proper sun protection later in this chapter.

Before we review some other quick fixes for your acne crisis, it must be clear what things you must avoid to clear up your acne faster.

We already spoke about the importance of avoiding sun for other skin problems; well, it is true for acne, too. Sun will inevitably worsen acne, usually two weeks later, with deeper more inflamed pimples that are trapped under a new layer of sun-damaged skin cells. Don't be fooled by the temporary relief from acne you may believe you get after being out in the sun. This is a transient anti-inflammatory effect that we know UV radiation has, but the harm of worse acne later outweighs any good.

In recent years, dermatologists figured out that acne may be triggered and worsened by high sugar diets and certain forms of dairy. I advise you avoid refined sugars, skim milk, and lactose-rich dairy and, instead, go with a low glycemic plant-rich diet. Dairy is acceptable, if it is in moderation and is lactose-free or very low lactose. You may need to start reading food labels to learn which foods are safe.

The following is my list of acne triggers to avoid or things that may make your acne worse: improper face cleansing, stress, hormone changes, over-application of occlusive moisturizers, occlusion of the skin, heredity (family genetics), high glycemic diet (sugars, carbohydrates), skim or fat free milk, certain topical oils (see Certain Oils section below), whey protein supplements, steroids, medications like Lithium, and certain hormonal contraceptives (Mirena, Depo-Provera, Norplant). While one cannot avoid heredity, the other triggers can be controlled or avoided pretty easily.

Spinning Brushes

I caution about these devices as they have very limited proof that they are helpful to our skin. I have seen in my dermatology practice that many people with acne try those brushes, regardless of the brand and get no improvement or worse acne. The concern is that the brush bristles may inflame the skin more, which can clog the pores more and give more acne. The brush bristles may retain dirt, bacteria, and other microbes and just grind them deeper in our skin. Knowing that we all have normal bacteria, yeast, and even mites living on our healthy skin, the thought of grinding them around is pretty gross. I would like to see more controlled studies employing these devices. Their original purpose was to try and simulate microdermabrasion treatments for home. Microdermabrasion is a light exfoliating skin treatment done by aestheticians in spas. There is very limited data to support that microdermabrasion is effective or helpful for any skin disorders. Such treatments are typically too shallow to correct skin scars or most skin discolorations. Certain types of acne where the inflammation is deep in the skin are unlikely to benefit from these superficial treatments.

Makeup Sponges/Brushes

When you are acne-prone, be sure to disinfect makeup sponges, brushes, or other applicators. The cold sterilization or herbicide used in hair salons or 70% alcohol or bleach would work. All these tools may collect dirt and microorganisms (yeast, bacteria, and mites) from our skin and the air between uses. If you are applying makeup with your hands, be sure and wash your hands prior to starting.

Certain Hormone Medications and Steroids

While most birth control medications are helpful for acne in women, there are certain types that are not. A review of the birth control for acne research has shown that the following forms of hormonal contraception actually worsened acne in some users: Depo-Provera, Norplant, and Mirena IUD. There are currently three oral contraceptives approved to treat acne: ortho-tricycline, Yaz, Estrostep, as well as their generic equivalents. It is also well known that ingesting (exogenous) steroids or supplements containing steroids will likely worsen acne.

Certain Oils, Fats, and Other Additives in Some Skin Products

Some ingredients in skin products and cosmetics should be avoided as they are considered by dermatologists to be comedogenic or acne-producing.

- Isopropyl isostearate – found in some bronzers
- Cocoa butter – found in moisturizers
- Jojoba oil – found in moisturizers
- Myristyl lactate – found in moisturizers
- Stearic acid – found in moisturizers
- Isopropyl myristate – found in sunscreen
- Octyl palmitate – found in sunscreen
- Corn oil – found in powder makeup
- Lanolin, Lanolin alcohol – found in skin creams and cleansers
- Vegetable oils in vitamin E capsules

Now, what do we do with this information? I realize these chemical names are not memorable and outright boring. You could, at least, check your skin products and verify that they do not contain large quantities of any of these. Another important point to remember is just because it is not listed here, it does not mean the chemical is not comedogenic or acne-causing. Unfortunately, there is limited data on this topic of what chemicals in skin products could give acne. Therefore, when a new formulation or new product becomes popular like coconut oil and other oils recently, I would caution to test it first on small areas of the skin. In addition, trendy skin product ingredients do not always have good medical research to support that they work well on our skin as they may in our food or for other uses. Some common oils and ointments, like mineral oil and white petrolatum, are typically not acne-causing but may cause acne if overused and applied for more than one week on the same place on an acne-prone area like the face.

Sun and Acne

In the past, some dermatologists would advise their patients to get a little sun to calm their acne. Sun exposure for acne is not recommended by dermatologists today because we better understand that the hazards of too much ultraviolet light in sunshine outweigh any small benefit. While it is true that ultraviolet light suppresses inflammation in skin problems including acne, this benefit can be isolated and used in a safe way to treat your skin with the new acne in-office and home low-level light devices. Unfiltered sunshine is carcinogenic or cancer-causing but we believe the low-level light is not. There are other hazards of the sun while treating your acne, beyond the carcinogenicity.

Another hazard of getting sun while treating acne, is that the sun can dry out the already dead skin cells or kill some that were not dead yet, which creates a thicker dead skin cell layer. This thicker dead skin cell layer may in turn clog more pores, resulting in more acne.

Many acne medications are sun-sensitizing as they may exfoliate the dead skin cells. This can significantly increase the risk of a sunburn or brown discoloration from the sun, while treating your acne.

So hopefully you are hearing my message clearly that sun is not good for acne-prone skin or for skin that is being treated for acne. Never go outside or sit near a window for more than ten minutes, without sunblock or sun protection while treating your acne. If you are concerned about vitamin D, then you should be able to get that adequately from diet and/or supplements.

Lasers, Lights, and Devices

The first-line treatments for the type of acne that does not respond to home remedies and is more moderate or severe are prescription topical and oral medications prescribed by your dermatologist. Spa, laser, and light treatments are effective for most forms of acne but they range in price from $40 to thousands of dollars. These treatments are not usually covered by your health insurance plan, so you will have to pay upfront for them. Many times, these treatments will help improve the acne faster if done in combination with the prescription treatments. In addition, spa, laser, and light treatments may be used as an alternative to prescription topical and oral medications. This can be helpful where there is an allergy or intolerance to a prescription. Continue reading to hear more details about the laser, light, and spa treatments that are typically helpful for acne.

At medical spas and some medical offices, a master aesthetician can do treatments that are helpful for your acne such as chemical peels, acne extraction (pimple popping), and some gentle light and laser treatments. Chemical peels are usually meant to exfoliate the skin, which can clear out pores, fade discolorations, and smooth the skin. Unless done by a physician, the chemical peel effects will be mild. Gentle chemical peels may be repeated every two to four weeks for full benefit. Some physicians will offer stronger chemical peels like 'Jessner's' or 'TCA (Trichloroacetic acid),' which can exfoliate, fade discoloration, and smooth the skin more aggressively. This is helpful for more severe acne and acne scars. For the most severe scars, the doctor may recommend subcision and laser resurfacing.

Many of my patients ask me what the best cosmetic treatment would be for their skin. There are often many good treatment options and the choice can be very individualized. To choose the best one, I recommend you and your dermatologist discuss the pros and cons of any particular treatment and guide you in choosing which treatment is best for you.

Acne extraction (pimple popping) is best done by trained hands, such as with a master aesthetician, nurse, or physician. If not done properly, you may increase your risk of discoloration or scarring. I have seen lots of people take matters into their own hands when it comes to popping the pimple and they go on to develop infection and or bad scarring. It's usually because they squeezed and popped too aggressively. If a pimple becomes infected, it may fill with pus, enlarge, and become red and painful. At this time, it would be considered an abscess, and should be drained surgically by a professional. After drainage, you may be prescribed antibiotics to treat infection. A dermatologist may also recommend injection of an inflamed pimple with an anti-inflammatory steroid medication like Kenalog (triamcinolone).

Low level light, also known as red, blue, and infrared light may improve acne. These treatments are most effective with the larger in-office lamps. There are some home light devices that offer mini alternatives to the in-office lamps and are also helpful. In general, the home mini lights require more treatments to achieve the same improvement as the larger in-office light.

Intense-pulsed light (IPL) treatments (photo-facials) are typically done in the doctor's office with either a nurse or physician. They are very helpful to calm inflamed acne and improve discoloration. Intense-pulsed light is not as helpful for texture problems like bumpy scars. The way IPL works is to improve acne through certain wavelengths of light emitted that are absorbed by unwanted colors in the skin. Red and brown discoloration can be targeted. One to three treatment sessions are generally needed for best results.

Lasers can be used to calm or improve active or inflamed acne as well as acne discoloration or scars. Some gentler laser treatments that require less healing time and repeat treatments for best results may be done by a nurse or physician assistant in a dermatology or plastic surgery practice. There are laser treatments that are more intense and produce more dramatic improvement. They require more healing time but fewer repeats and are usually performed by the physician. There is no perfect cure for acne scarring at this time but the laser treatments can be quite effective at improving the scars. Since there is no perfect fix or cure for acne scarring, it is important to prevent acne scars with proper treatment and identification of severe cystic scarring acne. If you think you have this kind of acne, you should see a dermatologist as soon as possible.

Shrinking the Pores

Before you get too excited, there is no surefire way to shrink one's pores but there are ways to improve the pores. Treatments like nose strips do not shrink pores, but may temporarily clear them out so they are less visible. The pores are likely to refill one to two weeks later. Treatments with chemical peels also may temporarily clean out clogged pores but will not shrink the pores in any lasting way.

Topical retinoid medications used to treat acne will help reduce sebum (oil) from pores, exfoliate, or shed dead skin cells from the skin which is all helpful for diminishing the size of pores during treatment but is not permanent.

Some newer radiofrequency and laser skin treatments are suspected as being capable of shrinking pores, maybe, even long term, but there is not enough clinical research data to prove their power yet. There is hope that within the next five to ten years these treatments will be better understood and studied and a cure for large pores will be discovered.

Body Acne and Boils

When acne spreads beyond the face, it can be challenging to control. It is not practical to hand-apply medicines to all locations on the body. Where the acne is located, it can, sometimes, tell us about the origin and how to best treat it.

Fine and small pimples on the mid chest and mid upper back are seen with pityrosporum or yeast acne. I discussed this entity and how to check for it earlier in the 'Things That Look Like Acne but Aren't' section of Chapter 5, so go back and review as needed. Larger and inflamed pimples on the chest, shoulders, and back are seen with hereditary cystic scarring acne, and sometimes with hormone irregularities. Men who take oral steroids and women who have polycystic ovarian syndrome may get this kind of acne. This severe type of acne may require an intense oral treatment and may best be managed at the dermatologist's office.

I have seen people with body acne that resolved simply by stopping or minimizing sugar in their diet. Present research confirms a link between high sugar diets and more acne but not specifically body acne, yet. Despite that, I have seen in my practice poor diet associated with body acne. In addition, boils are associated with obesity and the insulin resistance seen in type II diabetics, polycystic ovarian syndrome, and metabolic syndrome.

Boils can be managed with antibacterial cleansers like chlorhexidine, low glycemic diet, and exercise to reduce friction in skin folds. In addition, an oral zinc gluconate supplement has been shown to be helpful for some people with boils. I would take it twice a day as tolerated for recurrent boils. If your boils are more severe and they result in scarring, then you may have a disease called hidradenitis suppurativa (HS). HS is treated with the above measures I recommended for boils but if that fails, then you should see a dermatologist for prescription treatment.

Camouflage of Acne with Makeup

When you have acne and you wish to apply makeup, there are a few simple rules that one should follow to avoid problems or worsen the acne. These rules involve your choice of makeup and style of application.

First, choose a makeup that is 'mineral' as it will contain fewer chemical irritants. Second, apply makeup last: after skin medication, after moisturizer, after sunblock, and after serum. Third, apply your makeup in thin and small quantities, so as not to further clog your pores.

Try to clean your face gently twice a day; especially, if you wear makeup regularly. Do not wear your makeup to bed, as the more layers on your skin, the more to occlude your pores. In addition, makeup can attract and collect environmental debris, pollutants, as well as microorganisms throughout the day. All of this buildup can result in more breakouts or irritation.

Regarding technique of applying your makeup, if you have a stubborn and swollen pimple that you are struggling to cover, try an under-eye concealer. Under-eye concealers work very well to mask pimples. Try to match your skin tone, then go a shade lighter for best coverage. The correction pallets that contain violet, green, and yellow are helpful to cover big pimples, too, but require two layers where the first layer is the correction color and the second layer is your usual makeup base color. Finish with applying a light powder to set and protect your result. Do not cake on thick layers of concealer or base as this looks unnatural and odd and can attract negative attention.

If you would like to lightly cover up some blemishes but you are not accustomed to wearing makeup and need sun protection, then consider one of the tinted mineral sunblocks. They add a subtle tint of cover, regardless of your skin type and provide sunblock protection simultaneously. Men, who would like to camouflage their zits but do not feel comfortable using makeup, may be willing to try the tinted sunblocks.

Chapter 8

Quick Anti-Aging

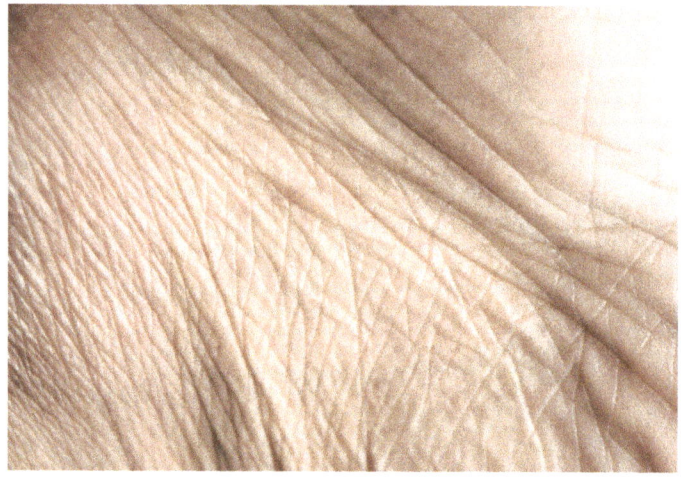

With aging, our skin loses healthy collagen, elastin, hyaluronic acid, water, and many other healthy structural elements resulting in wrinkles, sags, and hollows.

You are probably doubtful that you can fix your wrinkly and saggy skin in less than thirty days, but I will teach you the fastest fixes for aging skin that dermatologists know. Just because it is fast, does not mean it is not good, effective, or lasting.

Let's Begin with What You Can Do at Home

Avoid the three S's: sun, sugar, and smoke. Ultraviolet light from sun, sugar in your diet, and cigar/cigarette smoke have all been associated with oxidation and glycation which result in more rapid aging changes in your body and skin. Did you ever notice that fair-skinned people who grew up in very sunny places tend to have worse wrinkles?

Moisturizing your wrinkly skin every day, at least once a day, is helpful to instantly diminish the appearance of those wrinkles. Choosing the right skin products can be very frustrating as there are too many choices nowadays. Most importantly, it is the ingredients and not the name or brand that is crucial. Next, the product should be backed up with good scientific data showing the ingredients actually penetrate the skin and work. I will explain the most important, clinically-proven ingredients that you should select. Certain newer moisturizers contain lipids called ceramides, which are particularly helpful to smooth and soften the skin.

Some of the newer moisturizers also contain 'hyaluronic acid,' which is a water-loving and anti-aging ingredient. Once applied, it will absorb water so quickly that it instantly swells, smoothens, and plumps away wrinkles. Hyaluronic acid (HA) is the key ingredient in most lip plumpers and some eye wrinkle creams on the market. HA is also the leading ingredient in 'filler' treatments that are done at the doctor's office. HA is an important structural element in our skin that needs to be replenished to fight aging changes. So, products containing ceramides and hyaluronic acid are both moisturizing and rejuvenating. I will now discuss some other effective rejuvenating ingredients in skin products and how to incorporate them into your daily skin care routine.

Growth Factors

Some anti-aging serums and lotions contain a new and exciting ingredient known as 'growth factors.' Growth factors are needed for cells to stay young and healthy as they lose these growth factors with age. Some other names for them are: TNS, TGF Beta, GM-CSF, EGF, PDGF, oligopeptides, redox signaling molecules, and more. Some growth factor ingredients are touted to stimulate renewal of the skin cell's 'extracellular matrix.' Others renew collagen and elastin formation. There are so many growth factor products on the market right now that it is a little overwhelming trying to choose which one to spend your money on. To make matters worse, they tend to be very expensive. Despite their price, when you get the right one, they are worth the dollars and can be used sparingly to last. I recommend you go with brands that have controlled clinical research studies to prove their legitimacy and results. You can search for the brands on the internet and review, if there are clinical studies present. If your local dermatologist carries one of the brands in their clinic, then you can usually count on that brand having clinical studies. The best growth factor creams are more potent and will give some results within four weeks. Growth factor creams are nice in that they are moisturizing, not usually irritating, they are unlikely to cause allergy, and do not typically show sensitivity to sun.

Retinoids

Long before growth factors in skin creams, there were retinoids. Retinoids, like the most famous and original 'Retin A cream' and its followers like Tretinoin, Tazorac, Differin gel, adapalene, and Retinol are all anti-aging and will improve wrinkles with regular use. Retinoids have years of good science to prove they work well for anti-aging and are typically less expensive than growth factor creams but they tend to be more irritating and sun-sensitizing. It is not unusual to get a little redness, peeling, and itching when you are using or starting a retinoid. I recommend applying a moisturizer after the retinoid at bedtime and a sunblock before going outside. Despite the small drawbacks to retinoids, they are so effective that they should always be included in any anti-aging skin care regimen.

Antioxidants

With age and the environment, our skin cells get damaged by free radicals every day. Antioxidants neutralize the free radicals to protect our skin and are a crucial step to help maintain your anti-aging results. They are available mixed in your moisturizer and, sometimes, as serums or gels. Vitamin C is popular but some formulations may give acne. Just as with growth factors and retinoids, the best antioxidant skin products are from companies that do clinical research studies to prove their products work.

For faster anti-aging results at home, you can use a combination of the best home topicals. For example, you could apply a growth factor serum or cream, a retinoid cream, and antioxidant serum all in the same day. Usually you would apply the one that dries the fastest first and you would avoid layering too many creams, if you are acne-prone. Most of these creams are non-comedogenic where they should not clog pores but, sometimes, when you are layering a bunch you can get clogging.

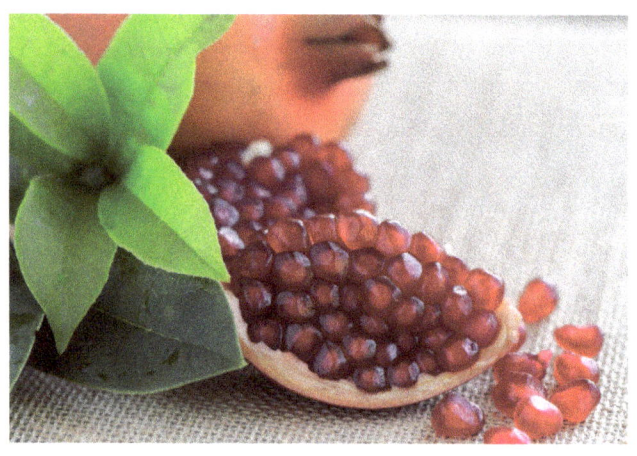

Oral Anti-Aging at Home

Most importantly, in order to have healthy, beautiful, and youthful skin, we must eat a healthy diet and stay fit. I recommend a low glycemic diet which is low in sugars and white-flour carbohydrates, rich in vegetables, low sugar fruits, and whole grains and just enough lean natural or organic protein. Sugar is believed to speed aging by a process called glycation, where our collagen and elastin in our skin gets glycated and loses proper function. If you have a history of getting a reaction or a rash from jewelry, then avoid nickel in the diet. Nickel is in a lot of things like nuts and chocolate, canned food, and more. To get a comprehensive list, you can look for a low nickel diet from the American Contact Dermatitis Society at contactderm.org. Mild to moderate exercise should be paired with your healthy diet for healthy, youthful skin. Inflammatory skin diseases like psoriasis have an increased incidence in obese people. We are still studying the relation between diet, exercise, and inflammation in your skin, but early data supports that a healthy diet and exercise may lessen skin inflammation and thus lessen skin disease.

There are limited studies on dietary supplements for the skin but there are some that have enough data to show they are safe and are likely helpful. The following dietary supplements are hypo-allergenic and may help improve the skin: zinc, vitamin C, vitamin D, omega-3 fatty acids, collagen peptides, turmeric, biotin, and milk thistle.

Quick Anti-Aging at the Office

Fading brown spots and evening out your skin tone can have a major impact on helping you to look younger. Psychology studies have shown that people, who have fewer brown discolored spots and more even skin tone, give the impression of being younger, healthier, and even, smarter. Be sure and review Chapter 3 as well for help with fading brown discolored spots on your skin.

In the office, brown and red spots can be faded quickly with IPL or BBL. These are light treatments that are usually safe and effective when done by an experienced cosmetic specialist like a dermatologist, plastic surgeon, or physician assistant to those doctors. When done at medical spas by assistants, these treatments may be muted and not as effective if you want rapid results. Some chemical peels are as effective as IPL and BBL but unlike these light treatments chemical peels cannot fade red discoloration and may not get deeper, stubborn brown spots as well. IPL and BBL treatments usually have a quick recovery and improvement time period of less than two weeks. Even one treatment done at the doctor's office will give nice results. Some people with more stubborn or thicker discolorations will need multiple treatments.

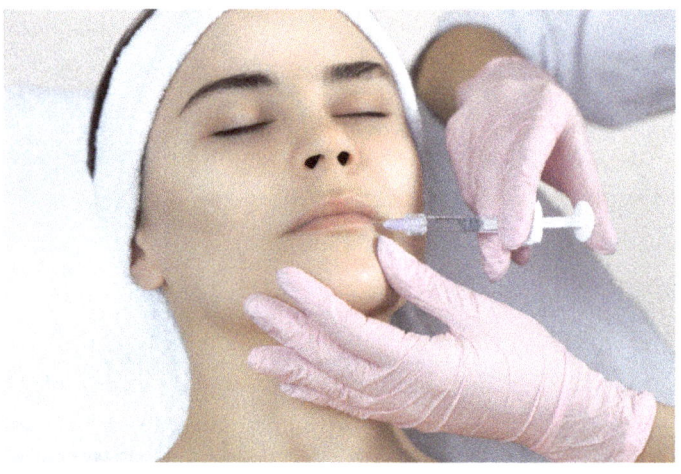

Filler treatments done at the doctor's office can produce quick results with instant improvement in moderate wrinkles, sags, bags, scars, and hollows. Filler treatments are needle injections done with or without local anesthesia. Recovery is rapid too, with just a week or less of bruising or swelling. If you are careful to avoid blood thinners in your diet and supplements for at least ten days before your treatment, you will have less bruising. The following are blood thinners that could be avoided before your filler treatment: aspirin, ibuprofen, vitamin E, fish oil, omega 3/6,

St. John's Wort, and garlic. Filler treatments can be done in small aliquots to see gradual results and will never look unnatural or fake with a skilled injector. Filler treatment is something that could be done three weeks before your event. I say three weeks to allow for any bruising and swelling to diminish and time for any small touch-up treatments which are rarely needed. Filler treatments with hyaluronic acid are very safe and hypoallergenic. Filler injection treatments may not be appropriate in people with certain autoimmune diseases. Filler products are approved for treatments in certain areas of the face, but skilled cosmetic filler specialists will sometimes offer filler treatments to off-label areas on the face. Off-label treatment is still safe when done by experienced cosmetic specialists like dermatologists and plastic surgeons. Complications from fillers are rare because the hyaluronic acid filler can be dissolved quite easily with an enzyme. Some treatable and usually temporary complications of fillers include: lumps, bumps, infections, and blood vessel blockage.

Botox and its sister products such as Dysport and Xeomin are neurotoxins that temporarily block the nerve to muscle signal, resulting in muscle relaxation. It lasts about three to four months. The doctor injects the Botox into the muscle to relax it, which, in turn, will smooth an overlying wrinkle. Botox is a temporary help for some wrinkles, mainly those on the brow, forehead, crow's feet, and lips. Botox can also be used to soften neck lines and sharpen the jawline. Botox can be a nice compliment to filler and may help maintain filler results. Botox is not for everyone. Sometimes the muscle relaxation can result in too heavy a brow or forehead, especially in older women. Botox is not recommended in people over 65.

For rejuvenating injections with either Botox or fillers, it is best to have a core cosmetic physician like a dermatologist or plastic surgeon do the treatment. There are a lot of doctors and nurses out there who attempt to inject and think it is easier than it is. This is why I believe we have lots of people with bad and unnatural results walking around. A good, honest injector will decline a person who asks for something inappropriate or likely to look unnatural and fake.

Non-ablative laser treatments, those that do not peel, can be done to rejuvenate with just one to two weeks recovery maximum and to have you ready within thirty days. These laser treatments are effective at stimulating new collagen and elastin for rejuvenation. There is an immediate glow after most of these treatments but the full improvement with new collagen and elastin may not be seen for a few months with repeat treatments. Recovery typically involves some blotchy red swelling of the face or treated areas for at least a week. Given the quick recovery and the early glow, it is reasonable to begin your first of two or three treatments even within thirty days of a big event.

Under-Eye Darkness, Bags, and Sags

Some of us have hereditary under-eye darkness or bags, even as teenagers. If we are fortunate as to not have these problems as a teen, it still may develop as an adult. Hopefully, you already know to wear sunglasses to protect your eyes from the aging effects and harms of too much sun exposure. Not only are your eyelids vulnerable to these harms, but your eye itself. UV radiation from the sun to the eyes can give cataracts, ocular degeneration, cancer, and more.

As far as choosing eye rejuvenating products, there are lots of eye creams on the market, so it can be quite confusing to select one. The best antiaging eye creams were clinically studied and shown to penetrate and do their work. The best anti-aging eye creams I have been able to find contain a combination of the anti-aging ingredients discussed earlier in this chapter: retinoids, growth factors, and antioxidants. Select an eye cream that has a combination of these key ingredients. There are some eye creams that instantly smooth fine lines by depositing an invisible fibrous, net-like support. These are clever and are convenient for a quick fix, but are not going to offer any lasting results. Hyaluronic acid eye creams are similar in that they can instantly smooth the skin, but it is a temporary side effect that may last only minutes to hours.

An excellent and fast way to improve under-eye darkness or bags at the doctor's office is with a tear trough filler treatment. Hyaluronic acid filler can be safely injected into the groove below the under-eye fat pad bag as well as into a dark hollow under-eye. The filler usually lasts about a year and with each treatment there is stimulation of new collagen and elastin in your skin, so less filler may be needed with repeat injections. This treatment can be done for adult men and women of all ages and will improve under-eye darkness, hollowness, wrinkles, and bags.

Saggy or Full Neck

At home you can attack a wrinkly and saggy neck with a neck firming cream. The good ones usually contain retinols, hyaluronic acid, and growth factors which I explained earlier in this chapter. Apply a neck firming cream one to two times per day.

At the doctor's office nowadays, there are a lot more choices than a good old neck-lift surgery. I still recommend a neck-lift for severe cases or for someone who prefers faster and more dramatic results. The radiofrequency, ultrasound, and laser devices all can result in significant skin tightening. Most of these treatments need to be repeated two to four times a month apart for best results but some improvement can be seen at one month. The Kybella injection dissolves fat in the neck with multiple treatment sessions but may not tighten saggy skin as much as these other options.

Some people are genetically blessed with prominent neck bands. Sometimes Botox can be very helpful to fix that. Botox blocks the nerve signal to the platysma muscle of the neck that creates those bands. Botox lasts about three to five months and can be repeated when it starts to fade. Platysmal bands, as they are called, can be pretty stubborn but can be dealt with surgically if one desires.

Jade Rollers

Jade roller devices that you can refrigerate have become hot under-eye anti-aging gadgets. I do see the temporary benefits they offer. The act of massaging is relaxing and meditative. By massaging your under-eye skin, you may push out lymph fluid and venous congestion that has collected overnight or after napping, and, thus, lessen under eye swelling and discoloration. Refrigerating the roller and making it cold before use may enhance these effects as the cold will constrict blood vessels reducing venous congestion faster. At this time, we do not know of any long-term benefit of the jade roller eye treatment.

Silk Pillows

Beware of gimmicky silk pillow products that claim it is better for your skin to sleep on a silk pillow. They are expensive, especially if 100% silk. There are no clinical studies to date that support the anti-aging or anti-acne claims regarding silk pillows. Maybe there will be in the near future. For now, the only reason that is proven to choose a silk pillow would be that it is softer and feels good.

Pre-Cancers, Actinic Keratoses, and Seborrheic Keratoses

If you are reading this and frustrated because you know you have pre-cancers, actinic keratoses, or seborrheic keratoses that have been diagnosed before on your face or elsewhere on the skin and you are doubting something quick can be done for those. Well, read on, as I promise to share the quick fixes for those.

Seborrheic Keratoses are those wart-like, sandpaper-textured, and barnacle-like skin growths that occur all over our skin in increasing numbers with age. There are some reasonable steps to improve them quickly. The fastest treatment would be a liquid nitrogen or laser treatment at the doctor's office but there are some helpful steps you can also take at home. Home wart remedies like: salicylic acid, oregano or lemon essential oils, and apple cider vinegar may shrink the keratosis and even cure small ones. Simple moisturizing of the keratosis is also helpful to improve their look. If you choose to do only the home remedies, then you may not see as dramatic improvement.

There are ways to clear up pre-cancers quickly as well. If you have lots, more than six or so spots, or your spots have blurred edges, then it may be reasonable to do what dermatologists call a field treatment with Blue or Red light at the doctor's office. This treatment is done in one day, an hour plus, and is often covered by your insurance plan. For severe cases, you may need to repeat the treatment two to three times a month apart but there tends to be a lot of improvement after the first treatment. Other than this convenient light treatment, for a field treatment, your dermatologist can prescribe a cream that can be used to treat pre-cancers at home. The most commonly prescribed creams to treat actinic keratosis (pre-cancers) are fluorouracil, imiquimod, and ingenol mebutate. Creams may take many weeks to complete their treatment and heal you. These treatments will cause temporary burning discomfort, redness, peeling, and swelling in the skin. The importance of curing the pre-cancers far outweighs the nuisance of the treatment discomfort.

If you have just a few spots, then it is reasonable to spot treat them at the doctor's office with liquid nitrogen. This would be faster than trying a prescription cream at home. A typical liquid nitrogen spot treatment for an actinic keratosis is usually healed within three to four weeks.

Chapter 9

Warts, Tags, and Other Skin Bumps

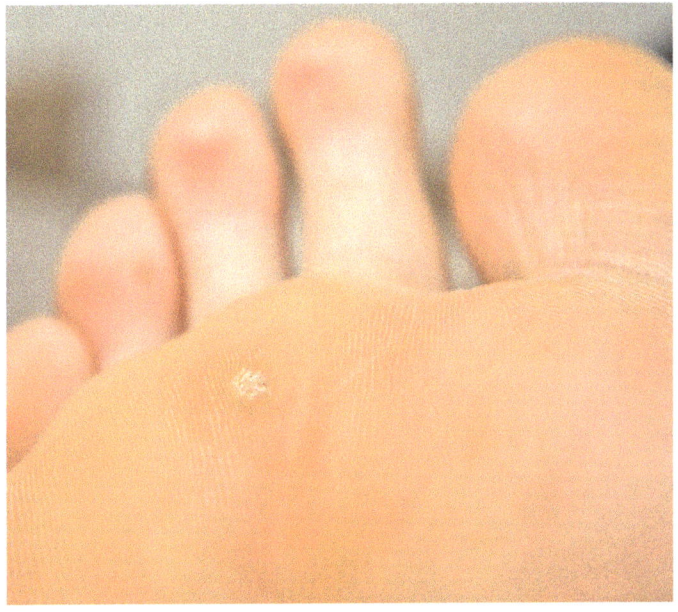

Typical plantar wart shown above

Yes, it is possible to fix warts and tags on the skin quickly, even at home. Before you get all excited and dive right into this, you need to verify that you have a wart or tag on your skin. Maybe you already were diagnosed by a doctor or you know from experience.

Warts are dry and hard bumps usually on dry skin areas that have brown or black speckles. They are caused by a virus and are contagious but are usually seen in people with dry skin and contact with others who have the virus. The warts spread with friction and rubbing of dry skin areas. Warts are very contagious and can be spread from one place on your skin to another if you are not careful. Controlling your dry skin is crucial to fighting warts quickly. If you fail to apply moisturizing creams to your affected skin, it will delay your healing and encourage growth and spread of the warts.

Maybe you have heard of treating warts with duct tape. Warts do not breathe, so duct tape does not work because it is suffocating the wart. That is nonsense that you may read on the internet. The dermatologist's explanation as to why sometimes duct tape will work to cure a wart is because the tape locks in the skin moisture very well and changes the environment around the virus so it is less favorable for the virus to invade and spread. So, the first step is to moisturize. Avoid picking, rubbing, or shaving over the affected skin or you may worsen and spread the warts.

There are wart remedies for sale at most markets that contain salicylic acid as the active ingredient. These medicines sometimes work but require persistence combined with frequent trimming of the wart for many weeks.

My favorite home remedy for warts that I have seen work with my patients, even with stubborn plantar warts, is oregano essential oil with or without apple cider vinegar.

Oregano essential oil smells quite strong, which is the main drawback. I wish it smelled like a pizza but, not exactly, it can sometimes smell more like hotdog water or a skunk. I recommend applying the oil with a cotton swab to the wart every night at bedtime, cover with a band aid, and repeat for as many days as it takes. Covering with a band aid will hopefully help mask the scent. If the wart is thicker, soak the wart in apple cider vinegar every morning before applying the oregano oil at night, and repeat this morning night routine until the wart is gone.

Another popular treatment that I have heard about from my patients is do it at home 'wart freeze.' These cold air canisters are weak and need lots of repeating to be only modestly effective. In the doctor's office, the first-line treatment is liquid nitrogen freezing. This is not always a quick method as it typically requires two to three treatments three weeks apart. Smaller warts are more likely to go away faster. Laser has not been shown to work any faster than liquid nitrogen. The doctor can prescribe wart remedies that work by boosting the skin immune system to produce a hive-like allergy reaction around the wart. They are helpful when other methods fail. Do not make the mistake of thinking you will cure the wart by cutting it off or having surgery. Remember warts are caused by a virus which you can't see with your eyes and it will be present in the bordering skin of the wart. This is why cutting it off does not work. I know there are some people who had their wart surgically cut off and got lucky as it did not seem to come back, but most of the time this method fails and you are left with a scar and a recurred wart.

Tags are dangly skin-toned growths that tend to occur in folds of the skin like the neck, armpits, and groin. They are triggered by friction, hormone changes, obesity, genetics, and possibly other unknown factors. I have seen women get them during pregnancy and others get them due to weight gain. Tags can be removed easily in the dermatologist's office. The dermatologist will usually clip or snip them off with sterile surgical scissors, apply a blood-controlling liquid, apply Vaseline ointment for healing, and cover with a band aid, depending on the location. Advantages to having your doctor do this procedure are: good bleeding control, sterile tools, and pain control with local anesthesia. Unless you have a bleeding disorder and worry about excessive bleeding, then you may be able to do this simple procedure at home. A curved manicure scissors that many of us have in our bathrooms can be used. I recommend sterilizing it with a flame or bleach prior to use. Clean your skin tag with alcohol prior to starting. After removal, the skin will need a few days to a week to heal. Applying Vaseline ointment twice daily to the wounds will help them heal. To be clear, I do not recommend removing a skin tag at home if you bleed easily or have a bleeding disorder, or if the tag has a base larger than two millimeters, as it may not be a tag as you thought.

Some people, especially darker skin types, may develop tag-like bumps on their neck and face. These are called 'Dermatosis Papulosis Nigrans' or DPNs by dermatologists. A famous example of these benign skin growths is the growths on the face of actor Morgan Freeman. They do not need to be treated but can be removed cosmetically. These are often removed by the dermatologist with either hyfrecator electro-cautery or laser. They are trickier to remove as there is a higher risk of leaving discoloration or scar from their removal in a darker skin type. I do not recommend trying to remove them at home because of the risk of discoloration and scar. If you can get an appointment for removal with the dermatologist, then plan on at least three weeks of healing and possible temporary discoloration for a few months afterwards.

Chapter 10
Closing the Deal

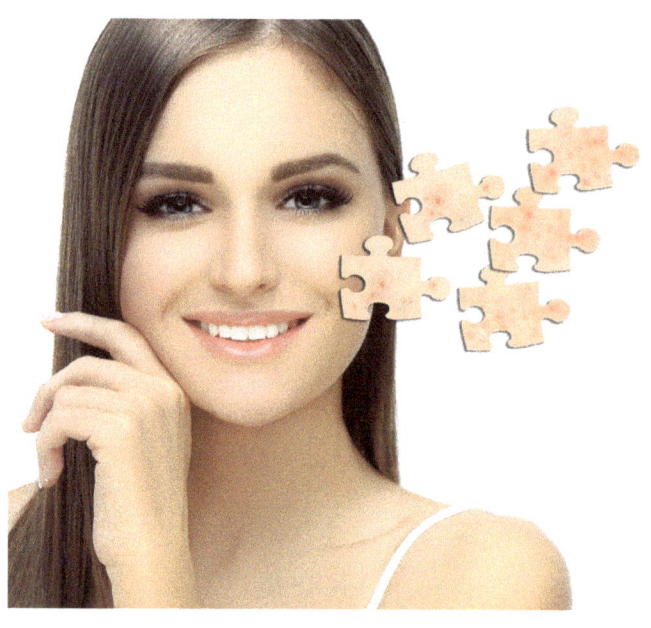

Hopefully, now you have put the pieces of your skin puzzle together, calmed your skin problem(s), somewhat, and started a new healthier skin routine. While your skin may not be perfect at thirty days, it may be improved and you're probably worried that at any moment it could go back to what it was. Here I will discuss some do's and don'ts to protect your good results and keep them coming.

Having nice skin has a little to do with genetics but there is a lot of environment that can be fixed to fix your skin. In simple terms, your skin environment includes the air (climate), water, health, diet, sun exposure, heat, and products you apply to it. Let's talk a little about the elements of your environment that can have a huge impact on your skin, health, and look.

Air

Dry air or climates tend to result in dry eczema or rash-prone skin. Along with dry skin, there is an increased risk of skin infections like common warts and irritant and allergic skin rashes. To combat dry air, you can have a humidifier in your bedroom or attached to your central air. If none of this is in your schedule or budget, then you may have to work at moisturizing your skin more than those in more humid climates.

Humid air or climates tend to result in better moisturized skin but sometimes over-moisturized skin is prone to yeast or fungal infections. In a humid climate, you may need to dry your skin better after bathing to avoid rashes and infections, especially in skin folds. Applying a powder to your skin folds, and other areas that get oily or moist may be helpful. Antiperspirants that are clinically strong may be helpful to apply not only on your armpits but to other areas like feet, inner thighs, mid chest, and under breasts. Just use the antiperspirant sparingly or you can over-dry and irritate the skin.

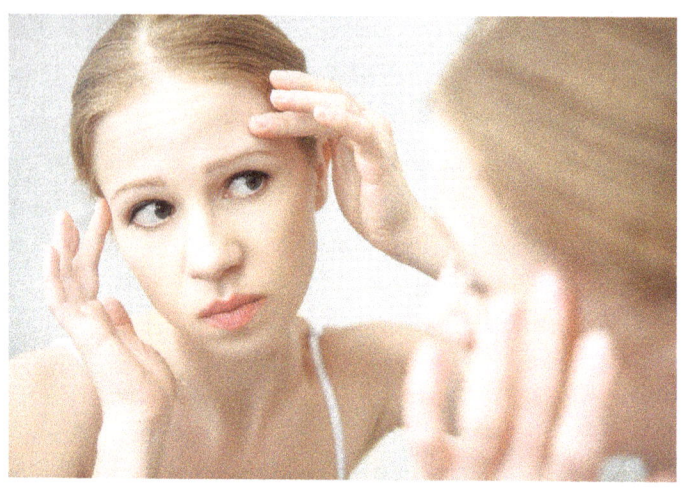

Water

Hard water contains minerals and is believed to worsen dry skin. There are studies that showed more eczema in populations with hard water. It is believed that soap surfactants will not rinse off the skin as easily with hard water and, instead, may clog pores worsening acne. In addition, the minerals in hard water remain on the skin as cations, which can form free radicals, which may age your skin faster by breaking down collagen and elastin. If you have hard water, don't panic, you just may need to use extra moisturizing and gentle soaps, cleansers, and emollients. If you do suffer from recurrent eczema or similar rashes, then you may want to consider getting a water softener in your home.

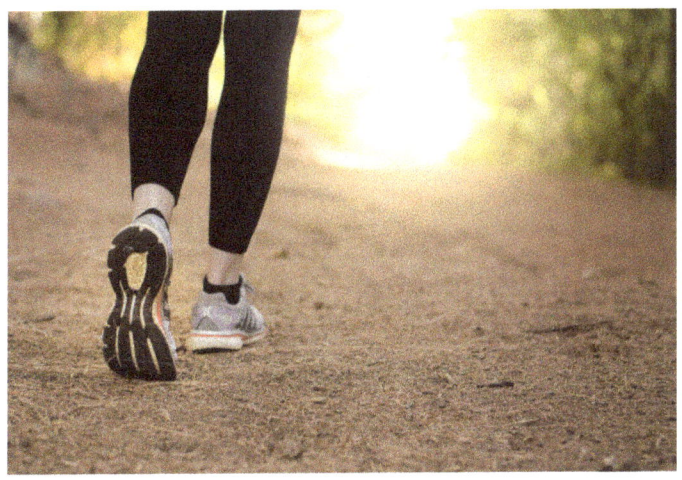

Health

In order for your skin to be healthy, the rest of your body has to be healthy too. That includes getting regular, at least, annual primary care doctor checks and doing any screenings that are recommended. In addition, for healthy skin, there should be no smoking, minimal alcohol intake, regular exercise to keep fit, and a well-balanced and low glycemic diet that benefits the skin.

When we are healthiest, our skin is said to glow. Some of us get trapped into trying too hard to get our skin to glow or be colorful and resort to tanning salons or heavy makeup. This can be counter-productive and, when overdone, may actually look unhealthy. Finally, the ultraviolet radiation we get in tanning salons is just as harmful, if not more harmful, as tanning outside in the sun. Cumulative tanning can cause deadly skin cancer. There is no such thing as a safe tan.

Unless it is the fake spray tans, those are ok. Just don't inhale them.

Diet

A balanced and low-glycemic diet is best for healthy skin. Low glycemic refers to when there is less sugar and carbohydrates. Avoid sugar and white flour carbohydrates that get converted to sugar more easily in our bodies. Eat more vegetables, fruits, whole grains, antioxidants, and omega 3 fatty acids. If you are wart-prone, try increasing your zinc intake. Zinc deficiency is associated with having stubborn and multiple warts. Make sure you get adequate vitamin D and B12 in your diet or supplements for healthy skin, nails, and hair. If you want to rejuvenate your skin, improve collagen and elastin, then try a collagen peptide supplement. There are a handful of studies that show these collagen supplements can help improve skin youthfulness. If you tend to have rashes such as eczema, psoriasis, or other inflammation in the skin, try a turmeric dietary supplement. Turmeric is anti-inflammatory and when taken twice a day in a potent supplement, it may benefit the inflamed skin. Recent science has shown that acne is worse in sugary or high glycemic diets. New studies have even shown that the gut bacteria in people with acne is different than normal. A healthy and low glycemic (low sugar) diet should protect most people from this imbalance in bacteria or you can see a gastroenterologist MD.

Sun Exposure

As I stressed in the Health section above, there is no such thing as a safe tan. Contour kits, bronzers, and spray or cream tans are safe but just might look funny, if overdone.

Those who live in a sunny region may have increased wrinkles, brown spots, and risk of skin cancer all at a younger age. If you live at sea level or below, you may not get vitamin D as easily from sun and should be sure to get it adequately in diet. I do not recommend sunbathing for vitamin D or ever, for any reason. It is a false myth that sun is good for acne. The sun does suppress our skin immune system briefly after exposure which gives the illusion that the acne is better but all the dead damaged skin cells left by the sun exposure clogs the pores and create more acne later.

Bottom-line, avoid the sun like the plague with protective clothing, hats, and mineral sunblocks that are applied evenly, and repeatedly every one and a half hour. The sun ages our skin with more force than any other factor.

Heat

I know I already said avoid sun like the plague but I will say it again for heat. If you tend to get redness (rosacea) or brown discoloration in your skin, avoid heat like the plague. Heat, also, can just inflame an already inflamed rash. Melasma and brown spots will worsen or darken with heat. If you have these heat-sensitive skin conditions, you must avoid hot tubs, saunas, steam rooms, hot showers, hot yoga, and other vigorous exercise in heat. A lot of people do not realize they have rosacea or a skin condition that worsens with heat and will join their pals in the hot tub, only to retreat back to their room with regret wondering why they look all blotchy and broken-out.

The End of Your 30 Days

If your thirty days are up and you are still freaking out because things are better with your skin but you don't trust that it will stay that way, now it is time to review and do inventory and continue the skin care that will maintain your good results.

For maintenance, it is most important to continue gentle daily cleansing, pH balance, and moisturizing. After that, remember to avoid any environmental exposures that have harmed your skin previously like the sun, wind, heat, hard water, poor diet, or stress.

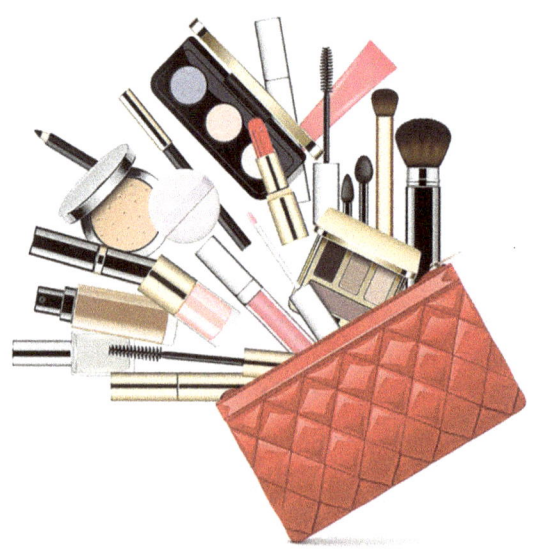

Many of the treatments that you may have started this month could be continued for further improvement and results.

If all else fails, then I have some urgent camouflage makeup tips for you.

Makeup is not just an art or fashion statement. When makeup is done well, it not only can hide flaws but can enhance youth, beauty, well-being, and health, all at once. When it is overdone or done distastefully, it can do the opposite. Unfortunately, many people do not recognize when they have crossed the line and overdone it. I am not going to instruct you on all aspects of skillful makeup application as that would defeat the purpose of urgency and haste when your goal is to be ready for an event within thirty days. I will offer some practical tips and tricks for anyone applying makeup. Even if you have a shaky hand, or you lack an artist's eye, you still can get good results with knowledge of some basics about makeup.

Makeup should be applied after moisturizer and sunblock for best results. I recommend contouring with a cream or powder base to highlight upper cheeks, mid and tip of nose, lateral brows, and temples. Contrary to some contouring makeup kits, do not darken the temples when over 35, as you will just accentuate hollowness and aging changes.

Avoid applying makeup too thick or it will give an odd and artificial appearance to your look. When trying to camouflage a pimple, discoloration, or a scar, always go with a cover stick color slightly lighter than the color you are trying to mask. Cover sticks or under-eye concealers tend to provide thicker coverage than liquid cover up. The contour kits as well as the yellow/green/violet correction palettes can be very helpful for camouflage. Yellow or green can cancel out purple and red. It is best to put only thin layers of these types of camouflage makeup to avoid distortion. After applying the coverage, it is best to set with a light powder that matches your foundation color or if you desire a tan look, then choose a powder with a tan hue.

Try to verify your makeup in multiple types of lighting such as natural, fluorescent, or soft. Also try to check your look with a loved one or friend who will be honest. Makeup should not be too visible or it will look odd and repel, rather than attract. Remember how you have reacted when someone with too much makeup walks in the room. You stare but not because they are attractive, rather because you are shocked and fascinated by how odd. There are psychology studies on beauty that show how people will not trust a person who looks odd or unnatural.

When choosing makeup base or foundation colors, try to match the makeup to both your face and neck skin tones together. You don't want a different shade on your face than your neck. Some people do have less color or tan on their face and they may want to choose a color that matches their neck. It is best to have the same tone from face to neck. When choosing blush and eye shadow colors, consider your overall tones between your hair and your eyes and skin. Brighter and contrasting colors will attract more attention and should be chosen carefully and sparingly.

I hope that at this conclusion of the book you have gained some valuable knowledge to help you maintain healthy and attractive skin.

www.ingramcontent.com/pod-product-compliance
Lightning Source LLC
Chambersburg PA
CBHW040108180526
45172CB00009B/1276